Medical Entanglements

Medical Entanglements

*Rethinking Feminist Debates
about Healthcare*

KRISTINA GUPTA

RUTGERS UNIVERSITY PRESS
NEW BRUNSWICK, CAMDEN, AND NEWARK,
NEW JERSEY, AND LONDON

Library of Congress Cataloging-in-Publication Data

Names: Gupta, Kristina, author.
Title: Medical entanglements : rethinking feminist debates about healthcare /
    Kristina Gupta.
Description: New Brunswick : Rutgers University Press, 2019. | Includes
    bibliographical references and index.
Identifiers: LCCN 2019007531 | ISBN 9781978806597 (pbk. : alk. paper)
Subjects: | MESH: Health Services Accessibility | Personal Autonomy |
    Feminism | Health Services for Transgender Persons | Healthcare
    Disparities | Bioethical Issues | United States
Classification: LCC RA564.85 | NLM WA 300 AA1 | DDC 362.1082—dc23
LC record available at https://lccn.loc.gov/2019007531

A British Cataloging-in-Publication record for this book is available from the British
Library.

♾ The paper used in this publication meets the requirements of the American National
Standard for Information Sciences—Permanence of Paper for Printed Library Materials,
ANSI Z39.48-1992.

www.rutgersuniversitypress.org

Manufactured in the United States of America

This book is dedicated to my son, Gabriel Castro-Gupta

Contents

Medical Entanglements

CHAPTER 1

Introduction

NO SAFE GROUND

This is a book about feminism and medicine in the United States. It is also a book about messiness, complexity, complicity, and irresolvability.

More than a decade ago, in connection with my interest in contemporary asexual identities, I started thinking about drug "treatments" for female sexual dissatisfaction (i.e., "female Viagra"). These interventions had been actively opposed by a group of feminist activists and scholars. Some feminist scholars had gone so far as to testify to the U.S. Food and Drug Administration (FDA) in opposition to these drugs (Tiefer 2006). Thus, when I began analyzing these interventions, I felt compelled to articulate my stance on them, and the choices seemed, at least to me, rather stark: for or against. On one hand, I was persuaded by feminist critics who argued that these "treatments" were developed primarily to increase drug company profits and that they inappropriately pathologized women's sexuality while ignoring social causes of sexual dissatisfaction (see, e.g., Tiefer 2006). On the other hand, I was persuaded by arguments that women have the right to experience sexual pleasure, if they want it, and thus should have the option to pursue pharmaceutical solutions (however imperfect) to sexual dissatisfaction (see, e.g., Nappi et al. 2010).[1] The more I thought about the issue, the more complicated it became. For every argument I added to the "for" column, I could add a counterargument to the "against" column and vice versa. As a result, I threw up my hands in temporary defeat and placed the project on the backburner, convinced that I would eventually be able to determine the "right" answer to the question once I had acquired the proper theoretical tools.

However, in the intervening years, I have read about or witnessed a similar kind of back-and-forth occurring over a number of different medical interventions. In these instances, in response to the promotion of a specific medical intervention, feminist, antiracist, queer, and/or disability studies scholars and activists offer a powerful critique of the normalizing tendencies of medicine and of its gender, race, class, and ability biases. In turn, medical professionals, patients, activists, and/or scholars respond with a defense of the intervention, arguing that the intervention could alleviate the suffering of some people. And the back-and-forth continues.[2] Sometimes, these discussions provoke heated feelings on both sides—the critic feels that her nuanced position is misrepresented or the patient seeking intervention feels that her lived experience of suffering is ignored. I have also witnessed a similar kind of back-and-forth occur in the classroom, as students struggle to reconcile their distaste for normalizing medical interventions with their reluctance to deny these interventions to those who seek them.

After much reflection, I have come to believe that there is often no "right" or "wrong" answer in these cases and no theoretical apparatus that can lead us to one "correct" position. Rather, I believe these debates are reflective of the broader sociopolitical reality—a reality riven with systems of inequality, including sexism, ableism, racism, classism, heteronormativity, settler colonialism, ageism, and more—such that both positions are, in fact, true (and false). It is the case that mainstream medical interventions, in the vast majority of cases, have been developed specifically to promote normalization and are used in the service of normalization. Here I rely on scholar Kim Hall's definition of normalizing technologies:

> These myriad, mutually reinforcing techniques of normalization subject bodies that deviate from a white, male, class privileged, ablebodied, and heterosexual norm. Seemingly unrelated technologies such as orthopedic shoes, cosmetic surgery, hearing aids, diet and exercise regimes, prosthetic limbs, anti-depressants, Viagra, and genital surgeries designed to correct intersexed bodies all seek to transform deviant bodies, bodies that threaten to blur and, thus, undermine organizing binaries of social life (such as those defining dominant conceptions of gender and racial identity) into docile bodies that reinforce dominant cultural norms of gendered, raced, and classed bodily function and appearance. (Hall 2002, vii)

Individual medical interventions are also developed within a broader context of (bio)medicalization, or the process by which more and more human problems and conditions have come to be defined and treated as medical problems and thus subject to medical study, diagnosis, prevention, treatment, and/or management. While contradictory in its effects, (bio)medicalization generally increases the power of biomedicine as an institution of social control (see Conrad 2007; A. E. Clarke et al. 2003). Individual interventions are also developed within the broader context of neoliberal capitalism, with its drive to place more and more responsibility on the individual to maximize their own health and productivity without public assistance (see Rose 2007; Rabinow and Rose 2006; Petersen and Lupton 1996; C. Roberts 2006). Finally, individual technologies of normalization have the power to shore up the broader system by increasing its legitimacy, mitigating the worst of its negative effects, and draining away discontent that might otherwise have been mobilized to support more radical political projects.

And yet, it is also the case that, in a white supremacist capitalist patriarchy, normalization can be a survival strategy, it can alleviate suffering (including the suffering caused by the system in the first place), and it can make bodies, minds, and lives more livable (more on livability later). In addition, while the majority of users will generally employ mainstream medical interventions in the service of normalization, in many cases, a minority of users will appropriate these interventions in the service of more subversive, nonnormative, or even queer ends. It is also the case that while normalizing technologies are often imposed on members of marginalized groups, access to medicine is also stratified via class and race lines, and thus members of marginalized groups may not have access to the very technologies that are being used by dominant groups to make their own lives more livable. An example of this comes from the scholarship on (in)fertility— Bell (2009) points out that, in the United States, infertile middle- and upper-class (usually white) women face pressure to use fertility interventions to achieve the socially expected role of biological motherhood, but infertile low-income women (often women of color) usually have no or limited access to fertility interventions, even when they desire them (Bell 2009).[3]

Thus, my intervention in this book is an analytical one—to show that, because of systemic inequality, many, if not all, mainstream medical interventions will simultaneously reinforce social inequality and alleviate some individual suffering. There is no way to think ourselves out of this conundrum; the contradictions are a product of unjust systems, not muddled thinking. Only a total transformation of the society in which we live could lead to the production of medical interventions that alleviate suffering without reinforcing social inequality.

My assertion that medical interventions will both reinforce social inequality and relieve individual suffering is a statement about *what is*, and much of this book is devoted to providing evidence for this assertion. This analytical insight about *what is* leads to both political/ethical and policy/practical implications. Ethically, this insight suggests that if we chose "for" medical intervention, we are supporting inequality (and the attendant suffering that comes from inequality), and if we chose "against" medical intervention, we are denying some people a way to alleviate their suffering (including suffering produced by current systems of inequality). In other words, both positions reduce and produce suffering.

In addition to offering an argument about *what is*, this book ventures into the somewhat more fraught terrain of offering an argument for *what should be* or, perhaps more accurately, for what feminist scholars and activists should do in response to the contradictory effects of medical interventions.[4] I suggest that we may have to accept that there is no ethically uncompromised position and that the ethicopolitical status of medical intervention may be irresolvable (indeed, accepting irresolvability may be the ethical position).[5] I am not arguing that the ethicopolitical status of all medical interventions is irresolvable—some interventions may be more clearly beneficial (casts for broken bones?) or clearly harmful (lobotomies for mental illnesses?)—but that, because of the imperfect world in which we find ourselves, the effects of a significant number of medical interventions will be good for some and bad for others, helpful by some standards and hurtful by others, beneficial at some levels and harmful at others, and, importantly, ultimately unpredictable, such that adopting a "for" or "against" position is not necessarily an appropriate response (although it may sometimes be practically necessary—in which case, one must simply take a leap of conscience and decide).

Practically, as unsatisfying as it may be, I suggest that perhaps the only option in a deeply unjust society is to allow individuals, in consultation with their communities of choice,[6] to decide for themselves whether to use a particular intervention, while working to implement some relatively simple safeguards to mitigate the worst social side effects of troubling medical interventions.[7] We can also work to create, as best as we can, a feminist democratic process[8] for deciding whether public or private insurance should cover the cost of particular interventions—strategies that are discussed in detail in the concluding chapter of this book. At the same time, I argue that our feminist, queer, antiracist, and crip activist energies should be directed not necessarily at opposing or supporting particular medical interventions but at addressing the broader sociopolitical structures that ensure that medical interventions are used largely in the service of normalization and working to ensure that all people, regardless of race, gender, sexuality, class, or ability, have access to the basic resources required to flourish.

To make this more concrete, in the case of (in)fertility interventions mentioned above, I would suggest that rather than taking a position for or against specific interventions, our feminist, queer, antiracist, crip political energies should be directed at dismantling compulsory motherhood (and especially compulsory biological motherhood) for middle- and upper-class white women while constructing a society in which low-income women, women of color, and gender nonconforming people are able to have children and raise them in a safe and supportive environment.[9] At the same time, while not opposing (in)fertility interventions per se, we might work to implement guidelines such that people who seek these interventions are also provided with information about alternative modes of family formation and connections to childfree solidarity networks.

I also argue that, as an ideal, we should work toward abandoning the framework of disease and "medical necessity" to justify medical interventions. This framework has led to a situation whereby a particular type of suffering must be framed as a disease (whether anyone actually believes it is a disease or not) in order to justify medical intervention and especially to secure public funding for or medical insurance coverage of a particular medical intervention. The disease framework simultaneously drives pathologization and reifies as "natural" the socially constructed distinction between health and illness. By presenting health and illness as natural categories, the framework of disease allows us to avoid acknowledging the reality that what gets defined as health and illness always depends on political and social decision making. In place of the language of health, disease, and "medical necessity," I propose using language such as "flourishing," "livability," and "fulfillment."[10]

The language of livability and "livable lives" comes from a variety of places. For me, it comes most directly from Judith Butler's discussion of precarity and livability. Butler argues that all human lives are precarious, but some lives are made more precarious and, in fact, some lives are not even recognized, and thus, when they are ended, they cannot be grieved. Thus, Butler argues that we must turn our attention to what conditions must be created in order to advance the flourishing of all lives or the *livability* of all lives. For Butler, livability is certainly about meeting basic needs for food, shelter, and physical safety, for example, but it is also about social recognition or social *intelligibility*. Butler writes, "When we ask what makes a life livable, we are asking about certain normative conditions that must be fulfilled for life to become life" (Butler 2004, 226; see also Butler 2006, 2016). The language of "livable lives" also comes to me more obliquely from disability studies—as discussed in Chapter 2, the Nazis described disabled lives as "lives not worth living," and thus, disability rights activists and scholars have insisted that disabled lives are worth living (they are livable) but can be made more livable through the elimination of ableism and the creation of a world that is designed to accommodate mind/body diversity (see, e.g., Hubbard 2013).

Of course, no term is perfect, and any term can be coopted or can acquire stigma if the phenomenon it co-constitutes remains stigmatized. However, at the moment, terms such as "livability" allow us to talk about different medical interventions (not "treatments") as promoting individual and/or communal flourishing, without needing to position anyone as lacking, deficient, or diseased in order to justify the use of a medical intervention. Leaving behind the framework of health and illness would also allow us to shift discussions about public funding for and insurance coverage of medical interventions away from doctors and medical researchers. In a transformed society, rather than relying on doctors and medical researchers to tell us what "counts" as an illness or as a "medically necessary" intervention (and thus is worthy of public support), a representative body of people could decide collectively what interventions should be publicly funded and what interventions should remain consumer goods, available for purchase by those who can afford them. Discussions about what interventions will promote livability are as fraught as discussions about what interventions are "medically necessary," but at least the altered language makes it clear that these are discussions about values, not just scientific or medical facts. Again, to make this more concrete, in the case of (in)fertility interventions, those seeking these interventions would no longer need to talk about infertility as a medical "disorder" (as is currently done in the United States) but rather could talk about (in)fertility interventions as making their lives more livable or as even contributing to their ability to live a fulfilling life. At the same time, as a society, we would need to decide through a feminist democratic process whether (in)fertility interventions should be publicly funded in all cases, some cases, or no cases.

IT HAS BEEN HERE ALL ALONG

The argument I am making here is not exactly a "new" argument. Most feminist, queer, and disability studies scholars who have analyzed medicine have emphasized the contradictory effects of medical interventions and the complicated relationship many of us have to medical interventions and practices of normalization more broadly. For example, in a classic piece on women and medicalization, Catherine Riessman states at the beginning of her discussion that there exists a consensus among scholars that medicalization has mixed effects and concludes her discussion by asserting,

> For certain problems in our lives, real demedicalization is necessary; experiences such as routine childbirth, menopause, or weight in excess of cultural norms should not be defined in medical terms, and medical-technical treatments should not be seen as appropriate solutions to these problems. For other conditions where medicine may be of assistance, the challenge will be to differentiate the beneficial treatments from those that are harmful and useless. The real challenge is to use existing medical knowledge selectively and to extend knowledge with new paradigms so as to improve the quality of our lives. (Riessman 1983, 17)

Although what I am arguing is in some sense the opposite of what Riessman states here (she does take a position against medical interventions for routine childbirth, menopause, and weight in excess of cultural norms and suggests that, while challenging, in general, we will be able to differentiate beneficial treatments from harmful treatments), her understanding of medicalization as contradictory in its effects and her call for both the limited use of medicine and a reimagining of its paradigms finds some resonance in this project. In a short piece, "Medicalization, Medical Necessity, and Feminist Medicine," Laura Purdy similarly discusses the contradictory effects of medicalization, both critiquing medicalization and pointing out that rejecting medicalization entirely can reinforce the dichotomy that Western society has created between nature and culture. She writes, "These points imply that women's health will be far better protected by political action than by medicalization. Does it follow that women's health and reproduction should be excluded from the medical realm? Surely not" (Purdy 2001, 255). As a third example, in "Cosmetic Surgery, Suspect Norms, and the Ethics of Complicity," Margaret Olivia Little explores the ethics of using cosmetic surgery to make women and African Americans more closely resemble male European standards of beauty. She argues, contrary to some in the medical profession, that cosmetic surgeons who perform these surgeries are, in fact, complicit with racist and sexist hierarchies. However, she suggests that there is some role for medicine to perform surgeries "even in cases involving suspect norms" (Little 1998, 175). At the same time, Little argues that surgeons who decide to perform these surgeries in order to alleviate patient suffering and pain must simultaneously fight against racist and sexist hierarchies. She writes,

> There is a limit to the suffering we require victims of the norm to bear before taking measures to escape that suffering, and health care professionals are sometimes the only ones who can alleviate that distress. Determining medicine's proper role in helping people meet suspect norms of appearance, then, is a complicated task, for there are two relations a physician must properly juggle—her relation to the individual patient, and her relation to the system of norms. . . . One must, if one participates in such surgeries at all, maintain an overall stance of fighting against the system. (Little 1998, 175)

Little's argument is similar to the argument I am making here, although she concerns herself only with the case of cosmetic surgeries and focuses on the moral responsibility of the physician. In addition, she seems to suggest that the subset of medical interventions involving "suspect norms" is limited, whereas I am suggesting that many, if not most, medical interventions raise these kinds of ethical and political questions. Still, her twofold position—of potential support for individualized interventions combined with active effort to dismantle systems of oppression—is compatible with the position I adopt in this book.[11]

A number of disability studies scholars have also adopted a nuanced understanding of medicine. While critiquing the pathologization of nonnormative bodies has been of critical importance, a number of scholars have also alluded to the complexity of the relationship between disability justice and medicine. In an early work in the field of feminist disability studies, philosopher Susan Wendell argues that social factors alone do not cause disability but that "the social response to and treatment of biological difference constructs disability from biological reality, determining both the nature and severity of disability" (Wendell 2013, 42). She continues, "We need to acknowledge that social justice and cultural change can eliminate a great deal of disability while recognizing that there may be much suffering and limitation they cannot fix" (Wendell 2013,

45). In addition, while she offers a searing critique of the cognitive and social authority of medicine, she also demands recognition for bodily experiences of suffering and, in some cases, the need for people experiencing physical suffering to distance themselves from their bodies. About medical cure, she writes, "Even people with disabilities who identify strongly with being disabled and have very happy, fulfilling lives might want to be cured, not for social reasons, but because they want to have less pain or physical or mental difficulty"; however,

> the widespread message that [people with disabilities] are not good enough until they are 'cured' places the self-respect of people with disabilities in conflict with any desire to be 'cured'. . . . Perhaps the best summary of my attitude toward 'cure' is this: I would joyfully accept a cure, but I do not need one. If this attitude toward 'cures' were taken for granted in my society, then the search for them would not be accompanied by insulting implications, as it often is now. (Wendell 2013, 82–84)

As another example, disability theorist Tobin Seibers supports what he calls "the theory of complex embodiment" in relation to disability—or the claim that society and the body are mutually transformative—and that disability can be the product of a disabling environment, or the body, or, in many cases, the interaction of the two. As a result, according to Seibers, "Some disabilities can be approached by demanding changes in how people with disabilities are perceived, others by changes in the built environment. Some can be treated through medical care. Other disabilities cannot be approached by changes in either the environment or the body" (T. Siebers 2013, 291).

This book also shares a particular affinity with Eli Clare's book, *Brilliant Imperfection: Grappling with Cure* (2017), which combines memoir with critical analysis to explore the ideology and practice of "cure"—which leads people to believe that the mind/bodies deemed "broken" by society are in need of "fixing." Clare traces the catastrophic effects of the ideology of cure on people with disabilities, in particular, both historically and in the present. As a result of these effects, for many years, Clare endorsed what he calls an "anti-cure politics." However, according to Clare, over time, his anticure politics were challenged, and he began to see cure as an incredibly contradictory phenomenon. Writing about his own effort to understand cure, he says,

> I couldn't tell any one story without being interrupted by a half dozen others. I landed inside a knot of contradictions. Cure saves lives; cure manipulates lives; cure prioritizes lives; cure makes profits; cure justifies violence; cure promises resolution to body-mind loss. I grappled through this tangle, picking up the same conundrums and questions repeatedly, turning them over and over, placing them side-by-side, creating patterns and dialogues. (Clare 2017, xvi)

As a result of recognizing these contradictions, Clare maintains his critique of the ideology and practice of cure and affirms his commitment to what he calls "brilliant imperfection"—or the nonnegotiable value of mind-body difference, while also acknowledging the benefit, or even necessity, of cure in some cases (Clare 2017). I find much in Clare's project that is similar to my own—although I followed the opposite trajectory of Clare from a generally procure politics to a place of deep ambivalence—we have clearly been grappling with many of the same questions and have come to many of the same conclusions.

Thus, it is certainly the case that (almost) all scholars writing about medicine and gender, sexuality, race, and/or disability have generally taken the perspective that medical technologies have both good and bad effects (and, indeed, this position might be viewed as simply "commonsense," although that term has been rightly troubled by feminist critics), yet we seem to repeat similar disagreements about specific medical treatments on a relatively regular basis. What I am contributing, then, is not the insight that many medical interventions have contradictory effects but the argument that many, if not all, mainstream medical interventions have or will have these contradictory effects (reinforcing inequality, creating suffering, and relieving suffering) *because* of the broader system in which they are produced and utilized and that these contradictions cannot be resolved analytically. What I hope to contribute, in addition, is a way, albeit imperfect, to move away from a "for" or "against" mentality in regards to medical interventions—specifically by accepting irresolvability and accommodation at the individual level (individuals deciding for or against specific interventions in consultation with their communities) while resolutely pursuing transformation at the macro-level (unjust social, economic, and political institutions and norms), while also recognizing that the two levels are intraconnected and that allowing for "individual choice" may make macro-change more difficult.

I make this argument through a case study approach, focusing on three medical interventions: transition-related care (sometimes referred to as sex/gender confirmation surgery or sex/gender reassignment surgery), sexuopharmaceuticals (such as Viagra and drug treatments for "female sexual dissatisfaction"), and weight-loss interventions (such as bariatric surgery). I chose these cases because each has generated some controversy and significant discussion by feminist scholars, activists, and the general public. Each case raises thorny issues about the role of social norms in the production of emotional, relational, and bodily distress, as well as the appropriateness of medical interventions in cases involving "suspect norms." At the same time, however, each case has its own unique particularities and reading them together creates a productive tension.

I start with transition-related care because, unlike in the other two cases, I believe there is no question that transition-related care can be life-saving for many trans people and can enable many trans people to live more fulfilling lives.

Yet, it is also clear that transition-related care can be a normalizing technology and there are significant problems with the way this care is currently conceptualized and delivered. As a result, the case of transition-related care in some ways requires us to develop analytical tools that allow us to hold these complexities together.

I turn to sexuopharmaceuticals next because I find their ethical and political status to be more ambiguous than transition-related care. It is clear that "erectile dysfunction" drugs like Viagra are primarily used to secure masculine heterosexual pleasure, at an individual and at a communal level. However, these drugs also, arguably, allow for new forms of sexual pleasure and are also employed in queer(er) sexual projects. The ethicopolitical status of drugs for female sexual dissatisfaction is even murkier; again, these drugs are likely to be used to increase the sexual availability of women to men but could also be used to facilitate female sexual pleasure. As a result, I argue that we cannot take a clear yes or no position on these drugs, but rather I advocate for a focus on transforming the broader norms about sexuality that structure the use of these drugs in such problematic ways.

I turn lastly to medical interventions designed to promote weight loss because I find these interventions most troubling from a feminist perspective. Drawing on insights from feminist and fat-positive scholarship and activism, I argue that it is clear that weight-loss interventions reflect and reinforce fat phobia. However, I argue that we must also combine feminist and fat-positive approaches with critical public health approaches that understand weight as socially determined and differentially distributed according to power and privilege. Combining these perspectives leads me to advocate, once again, for a focus on transforming aspects of our unjust society while understanding that medical or surgical weight-loss interventions may be the best option in some cases.

My hope is that the combined effect of analyzing these three interventions together will be to demonstrate that even in very different cases, it is often ethically appropriate to accept accommodation at the individual level while focusing on societal-level reform, with the recognition that the individual and sociostructural are mutually constitutive and that accommodation at the individual level could potentially undermine efforts to transform the structural level. Before introducing the structure of the book more fully, I next turn to outlining the theoretical tools I use to analyze each case.

THEORETICAL TOOLS

In general, this book adopts a feminist social constructionist approach to health, illness, and medicine. Lorber and Moore describe the goals of what they call a gender lens on health and illness as follows: "to show how gender, in conjunction with racial and ethnic identification, social class, and sexual orientation, creates different risks and protections for physical illnesses, produces different behavior when ill, elicits different responses in health care personnel, affects the social worth of patients, and influences priorities of treatment, research, and financing" (Lorber and Moore 2002, 3). In addition to this broad feminist social constructionist approach, this book draws on the following paradigms: *intersectionality, feminist science studies, queer studies*, and *disability studies*.

Intersectionality

Intersectionality is an analytical tool that has grown out of the work of black feminist scholars and activists (Crenshaw 1991; P. H. Collins 2005; Hancock 2016; McCall 2005; Cho, Crenshaw, and McCall 2013; Alexander-Floyd 2012). Although this analytical tool is itself contested, I take from it a fundamental commitment to understanding the intersectional nature of social categories (such as, but not limited to, gender, race, class, sexuality, and ability) and therefore the intersectional nature of identities that develop out of social categories (in other words, most individuals maintain multiple identifications, for example, a person might identify as a woman and as an African American) and the intersecting nature of privilege and oppression, such that an individual's access to resources and experiences of discrimination will be determined by the intersection of all of their social identities or by their location within multiple intersecting systems of power.

Importantly, social categories do not combine *additively* (e.g., a black woman does not have the experiences of a white woman plus the experiences of a black man) but instead mesh to produce qualitatively different experiences. Early formulations of intersectionality also critiqued "single-vector" (in other words, nonintersectional) analysis and activism for foregrounding the priorities and experiences of those members of a social group who have the most resources or privilege, while marginalizing members with the least resources or privilege— for example, feminist organizing has often focused on the needs of white women, while antiracist organizing has often focused on the needs of black men (Crenshaw 1991). In some ways, conducting an "intersectional analysis" is more of an aspirational ideal than an achievable goal, as it can be difficult to identify the social categories that are relevant in any particular situation (and, indeed, the ability to even "see" social categories that one does not belong to may depend on the extent to which these categories have been politicized); however, intersectionality remains the most important tool we have for understanding the complexities of oppression. According to Crenshaw, intersectionality allows us to analyze social problems more fully, shape more effective interventions, and promote more inclusive advocacy (African American Policy Forum n.d.). In this book, an intersectional analysis reveals the ways in which illness categories are always implicated with multiple systems of inequality and the ways in which access to health and healing are differentially distributed along lines of gender, race, class, and other social categories.

Feminist Science Studies

From feminist science studies, I draw three important insights. First, I take the insight that scientific and medical discourses, while purporting to be value free, are always "value laden"; in other words, they reflect the values of individual scientists and doctors, of scientific and medical communities, and of the broader societies in which they are located (Longino 1990; Keller 1992; E. Anderson 2004). Second, I take the insight that all knowledge, including both scientific/medical and feminist knowledge, is socially situated—in other words, it is shaped by the social location from which it was produced, and those producing knowledge from a minority perspective will often have greater insight into the society as a whole than those producing knowledge from a majority standpoint (Haraway 1988; Harding 1986, 2003; Alcoff 1993; E. Anderson 2004). Third, from feminist science studies, I take the overarching perspective that nature and culture or biology and society are not two separate entities but are always intertwined and co-constitutive. Donna Haraway has coined the neologisms *material-semiotic* (Haraway 1991a) and *natureculture* (Haraway 2003) to describe the imbrications of the material (biology, nature) and the semiotic (representation, culture, society). Drawing on the work of Haraway, Judith Butler, and Bruno Latour, among others, Karen Barad proposes the related concepts of *phenomenon* and *apparatus* to describe these imbrications. Every phenomenon that we observe in the world comes into view through a particular perceptual/cognitive apparatus. Both phenomena and apparatuses, according to Barad, are "intra-acting" material and semiotic entanglements. Apparatuses are boundary-drawing practices and are, themselves, phenomena (Barad 2007). It is from Barad's work that I take the term "entanglements" used in the title of this book.

Haraway's and Barad's work (among others) are useful for this project because they offer one way to think about illness and suffering as the product of cultural, social, and interpersonal factors "intra-acting" with bodies and biologies, with both sides of the culture/nature dichotomy determining the (always provisional) "outcome." In addition, they offer at least two ways to think about medical interventions as naturalcultural phenomena: first, medical technologies are themselves the product of both social/cultural norms and the possibilities/constraints of the materials out of which they are created and to which they are intended to respond (e.g., properties of neurotransmitters, centrifuges, assays, stomach wall linings, magnetic resonance imaging machines, and microscopes, to name a few). Second, they have naturalcultural effects—they are both social interventions and bodily interventions.[12]

Queer Studies

The third field from which I draw theoretical tools is *queer studies*. Again a contested field, queer studies has offered a critique of the ways in which the categories of "normal" and "deviant" sexual desire, activity, and identity have been constructed through operations of power, and yet, these operations of power have been rendered invisible in order to make these categorizations appear "natural." Expanding from a focus on sexed and gendered bodies, desires, activities, and identities, queer studies has interrogated the social construction of categories of normalcy and deviance more broadly (see, e.g., Butler 1990; Sedgwick 1990; Warner 1993, 2000; Foucault 1990; Puar 2007; Ahmed 2006; Ferguson 2003; Muñoz 1999). I use this strategy of analysis in my interrogation of health and illness categories as socially constructed categories of normalcy and deviance that appear natural to us, while also demonstrating the ways in which these categories reflect heteronormative assumptions about gender and sexuality. In addition, queer studies has offered an understanding of oppositional politics as subversion, parody, and creative appropriation (see, especially, Muñoz 1999; Butler 1990). For example, Carrie Sandahl describes "queering" as follows: "Queering describes the practices of putting a spin on mainstream representations to reveal latent queer subtexts; of appropriating a representation for one's own purposes, forcing it to signify differently, or of deconstructing a representation's heterosexism" (Sandahl 2003, 37).

This understanding of oppositional politics is useful in illuminating how a minority of users and communities appropriates medical interventions for their own purposes, often forcing them to signify differently and, indeed, using them to achieve nonnormative material effects. At the same time, queer studies scholars have emphasized that subversion and appropriation are never innocent political strategies and their effectiveness will depend on a number of factors, and some practices that appear "subversive" serve to reinforce certain forms of oppression. For example, Christian Klesse argues that while queer practices of body modification are often understood as subversive, "the pervasiveness of neo-primitivist influences in western non-mainstream body modification calls into question any attempt to frame these practices as transgressive in any unequivocal way" (Klesse 2007, 276).

Disability Studies

The final field from which I draw theoretical insights is disability studies. From disability studies, I take a number of insights about the pathologization of nonnormative bodies. According to a number of disability studies scholars, Western societies have frequently approached human mind/body variation through the lens of medicine—physical and mental states that differ from an idealized norm are often labeled disordered, doctors and medical professionals attempt to correct disordered mind/bodies (in other words, bring them into line with the norm) through medical and technological interventions, and people with these mind/body variations are stigmatized. This is the case even though, in many instances, the distress associated with a nonnormative physical or mental state is often the result not so much of the state itself as it is the result of social stigma, discrimination, and the fact that the built environment is not designed to accommodate these bodily variations. As noted above, Susan Wendell argues that "the social response to and treatment of biological difference constructs disability from biological reality, determining both the nature and severity of disability" (Wendell 2013, 42). Rosemarie Garland-Thomson offers the following definition of disability:

> What we think of as disability begins in bodily variation and the inherent dynamism of the flesh . . . disability is the body's response over time to its environment. Disability occurs when the shape and function of bodies come into conflict with the shape and stuff of the world. The discrepancy between body and world, between that which is expected and that which is, produces disability as a way of being in an environment. Put more poetically, disabilities are the etchings left on flesh as it encounters world. (Garland-Thomson 2012, 342)

Tanya Titchkosky offers an interpersonal definition of disability, writing, "When used to relate to people, disability is a form of perception that typically devalues an embodied difference. Some noticeable departure from the desired and expected is often taken as disability. . . . This orientation grounds the critical understanding that disability should be regarded as that which exists between people; one cannot be disabled alone" (Titchkosky 2011, 5).

Yet, while arguing that the medical model is often harmful to people with disabilities and rejecting the notion that disability inheres in the body or mind, disability studies scholars have also recognized that a complete rejection of medical approaches is not viable. Some mind/body variations do cause pain, which can be alleviated through medical approaches. Disability studies scholars have also argued that traditional activist critiques of medicalization can have at least three major pitfalls: first, often these critiques do not challenge stigma against ill people in general but simply try to move certain groups outside of the category of illness. Second, they often rely on the essentialist position that people should embrace or be true to the body and mind that they are born with and that efforts to transform the body or mind through medical and technological interventions are illegitimate. Third, they often lead to the policing of community borders—people who do employ medical or technological interventions are seen as in some way betraying the community. Thus, as a result, disability studies scholars have attempted to develop ways to critique the normalizing power of medicine, while also making room for medical approaches (Wendell 2013; T. A. Siebers 2008; McRuer 2006; Garland Thomson 1997). It is this multifaceted response to medicine that animates much of this book.

SOME NOTES ON SCOPE AND TERMINOLOGY

The scope of this book is limited primarily to ideologies and practices of medicine in the contemporary United States. This is the case because ideologies related to medicine as well as healthcare systems differ significantly in different countries. However, many of the broad arguments in this book may also apply to medicine and healthcare in other Western countries. In addition, as discussed more fully in the next chapter, Western medicine, particularly U.S. medicine, is, indeed, a globalized, colonial, and neocolonial project and thus touches on the lives of people all over the world. Thus, at some points throughout the book, the colonialist aspects of U.S. biomedicine are addressed.

It will be helpful to define here a few important terms used throughout this book that have not already been touched on. The first term that requires some elaboration is, not surprisingly, medicine. Practitioners and scholars have been arguing over the definition of medicine for centuries. Most would agree that medicine is some combination of science and art—in other words, scientific knowledge about the body, disease, and bodily interventions as well as practices (including diagnoses and treatments) that are derived from scientific knowledge, combined with the interpersonal interaction between a medical professional and a "patient" who comes to the professional for help with some kind of mind/body problem or issue (Marcum 2008). Medicine is also clearly an institution or set of institutions. In this book, medicine is used as a shorthand for Western medicine, which includes the knowledges, practices, and institutions that have developed in the West out of a tradition that dates back to the Ancient Greeks (Porter 2004). Contemporary Western medicine has incorporated, often in problematic ways, knowledges about the body and healing practices developed in other parts of the world—such as acupuncture—often describing these knowledges and practices using terms such as "alternative" or "complementary" medicine (Hollenberg and Muzzin 2010; Willard 2005).

Medicine does not have clearly defined boundaries, either in the world or in this book. It could conceivably refer to basic scientific research ("bench science") on the mind/body, multinational pharmaceutical companies making billions of dollars in profit, public health efforts to improve the "health" of populations instead of individuals, and practices undertaken by individuals without the involvement of any medical professionals whatsoever—such as dieting or exercise—if these practices are based on a medical understanding of the body and with the intent of promoting health or curing disease. Medicine can also refer to the ideology of medicine that infiltrates many aspects of Western society—which scholars have identified as the belief that sickness and health are material properties of the mind/body that can be understood and addressed through science (Wendell 2013; T. A. Siebers 2008; Clare 2017). Using such a broad definition of medicine runs the risk of obscuring differences between, for example, public health approaches that focus on the population level versus individual attempts to lose weight; however, using a broad definition also allows us to see connections between these various ideas and practices.

In part, a definition of medicine depends on a definition of health, illness, sickness, and disease, terms that are also hotly contested. There is no consensus about these definitions among laypeople, medical practitioners, or humanities and social sciences scholars who study medicine. In terms of health, at least two broad definitions coexist: health as the absence of disease and health as well-being and flourishing. Based on the first conception of health, medicine tends to be employed only to solve specific mind/body problems when they arise. Based on the second conception of health, medicine can also be employed to prevent disease or illness and to enhance quality of life. In terms of illness, sickness, and disease, different definitions abound—illness or disease is generally defined within medicine as a dysfunctional or harmful process within a bodily system. This definition is also held by some humanities and social sciences scholars who study medicine ("naturalists"). Many other humanities and social sciences scholars who study medicine argue that definitions of illness or disease always involve value judgments about what counts as a good life ("constructivists").[13] As noted earlier, in this book, I argue for setting aside the notion of disease altogether, and I discuss this issue more fully in Chapter 2 and the Conclusion. Thus, for now, it is enough to say that definitions of health, illness, sickness, and disease are always socially constructed and culturally specific (Boorse 1975; Kingma 2014; Jutel 2010).

Finally, in this book I use the terms "medical technology" or, more frequently, "medical intervention" rather than medical "treatment." In general, there are a wide variety of medical interventions, ranging from pharmaceuticals and surgeries to dietary changes and mindfulness meditation. When these interventions are intended to fix a specific problem or "cure" a disease or illness, they are usually referred to as "treatments," a term that generally has a positive connotation. However, queer, feminist, antiracist, and disability studies scholars and activists have argued that many so-called treatments are not necessarily positive and may even be harmful. Thus, I always use the term "intervention" instead of "treatment" because it does not have a necessarily positive or negative connotation—the value of the intervention is not predetermined as positive. I also do not distinguish between medical "treatments" and medical "enhancements," although some have argued that "treatments" (like antibiotics) are designed to restore the body/mind to "normal" functioning, whereas "enhancements" function to make already "normal" body/minds even better than normal. Instead, I agree with the many scholars who argue that there is no clear distinction between the two and the distinction, such as it exists, rests on the definition of "normal," which is always socially constructed (Daniels 2000; Wolpe 2002).

CHAPTER OUTLINE

Following this Introduction, in Chapter 2 ("Feminist Critiques of Medicine"), I offer a more in-depth overview of feminist critiques of medicine, which I organize into five categories: medicine as a *stratified* and *discriminatory* system; medicine as concerned with *profits*, not well-being; medicine as a system of *normalization*; medicine as *individualizing* and *privatizing*; and medicine as *alienating* and *displacing*. Given the size of this body of scholarship, I focus on offering brief summaries and a few examples of important works in the field. I then explore two possible responses to these critiques that have been proposed by scholars and activists: focusing on the agency of individual users in selecting particular medical interventions and working to clarify definitions of health and illness. Both of these responses offer valuable insights that I incorporate into my analysis of different medical interventions; however, I argue that neither is an entirely adequate response to the many problems built into the contemporary medical system.

In Chapter 3 ("Theorizing from Transition-Related Care"), I begin by introducing the scope of transition-related care and its history, along with a history of feminist, queer, and trans approaches to transition-related care. I then turn to outlining critiques of transition-related care as it is currently delivered before turning to a discussion of how this care might be reconceptualized and reformed. I conclude by highlighting the lessons that can be learned from trans-affirming approaches to medicine, arguing that trans activists and scholars who have worked on the issue of transition-related care have developed highly nuanced theoretical apparatuses that are capable of holding together a critique of the normalizing power of medicine along with an affirmation of the power of medical technologies to make some lives more livable and, in some cases, to promote flourishing.

In Chapter 4 ("Sexuopharmaceuticals"), I begin with an examination of sexuopharmaceuticals for "male" sexual dissatisfaction, primarily Viagra, tracing their history and feminist arguments for and against their use. I then turn to an examination of sexuopharmaceuticals for "female" sexual dissatisfaction, again tracing their development and examining their ethicopolitical status. I then turn to qualitative research conducted with asexually identified individuals. Asexually identified individuals have good reason to oppose sexuopharmaceuticals, especially those intended to increase sexual desire, as the existence of these drugs seems to suggest that a lack of sexual interest or attraction is pathological.

However, while most of the individuals interviewed were critical of sexuophar-maceuticals, they still felt that people should be able to access these drugs if their use would promote well-being. I argue that the asexually identified indi-viduals in this study offer the outlines of an ethically and politically responsible response to the contradictions embedded in the space of sexuopharmaceutical interventions. Ultimately, I argue that sexuopharmaceuticals, both as a broader discursive formation and as individual interventions into specific cases of sexual dissatisfaction, largely serve to promote and reinforce phallocentric and heteronormative sexual desires and activities; however, they can also be used to facilitate queer(er) desires and activities and, even in cases where they are not used "queerly," they may still promote well-being for some in a society not particularly well designed to promote sexual flourishing. Thus, I argue for directing activist attention away from directly opposing these drugs to work-ing to transform the broader society in order to create the conditions under which multiple forms of sexuality can flourish.

In Chapter 5 ("Constructing Fat, Constructing Fat Stigma"), I begin with examining traditional feminist/fat-positive and then critical public health approaches to weight. Feminist and fat-positive approaches to weight are useful for their critique of our cultural obsession with thinness and weight loss (and the consequences of this obsession for women in particular) and for the ways in which they challenge stigma against fat people and work to revalue fatness. How-ever, feminist and fat-positive approaches can miss the ways in which fatness is produced, in part, by public policies and corporate decisions that differentially burden women, people of color, and low-income people. Critical public health approaches to weight are useful precisely for their focus on the "social determi-nants" of weight. However, critical public health approaches are flawed when they heighten social pressure to be thin and/or increase stigma against fat people. Thus, I argue that combining the best elements of feminist and critical public health approaches to weight leads to a more complete understanding of weight as a political and social issue. I then use this combined perspective to reevalu-ate medical/surgical interventions to promote weight loss, with a focus on bar-iatric surgeries. Here I argue that medical and surgical interventions to pro-mote weight loss do not address, and may even exacerbate, the structural issues that lead to both fat-related stigma and discrimination and the differen-tial production of fatness; however, these interventions still may be a survival strategy in a unjust world and, compared to other individualistic interventions such as diet and exercise, may actually have some advantages from a feminist perspective.

In the Conclusion, I first make a general argument for replacing and supple-menting the language of "medical necessity" and "pathology" with the language of livability, fulfillment, and flourishing. Using the language of livability, fulfillment, and flourishing, I then offer a more general discussion of the threefold move argued for throughout this book: supporting individual decision making when it comes to medical interventions, establishing feminist democratic processes for determining funding for medical interventions, and engaging in praxis to create a more just society. Finally, I grapple with the issue of whether medical interventions are necessarily eugenicist.

CHAPTER 2

Feminist Critiques of Medicine (and Some Responses)

Although I have previewed a number of feminist, antiracist, queer, and crip critiques of medicine already in the Introduction, here I offer a more in-depth overview of these critiques, which I accept as foundational. This chapter is designed to introduce those who are not familiar with feminist studies of medicine to some of the key interventions made by feminist scholars and activists in this field.

I begin by briefly discussing the benefits of medicine for marginalized individuals and groups. My assumption (perhaps incorrect) is that most people raised in the West have been exposed to narratives extolling the benefits of Western biomedicine through media, schooling, and family experiences. Thus, I do not spend much time arguing for the benefits of Western biomedicine. I quickly turn to providing a short overview of intersectional feminist critiques of the history of Western biomedicine and then move to critiques of the contemporary system. Although the critiques of contemporary biomedicine are numerous and varied, while often sharing common themes, here I separate them into five categories for purposes of explanation: medicine as a *stratified* and *discriminatory* system; medicine as concerned with *profits*, not well-being; medicine as a system of *normalization*; medicine as *individualizing* and *privatizing*; and medicine as *alienating* and *displacing*.

After summarizing the most common feminist critiques of medicine, I then explore two possible responses to these critiques that have been proposed by scholars and activists: one, focusing on the agency of individual users in selecting particular medical interventions and, two, working to clarify definitions of health and illness. Both of these responses offer valuable insights that I incorporate into my analysis of different medical interventions; however, I argue that neither is an entirely adequate response to the many problems built into the contemporary medical system.

BENEFITS OF MEDICINE TO MARGINALIZED PEOPLE AND GROUPS

Before turning to a critique of Western biomedicine, I here acknowledge and honor the many ways in which Western biomedicine has benefited marginalized groups and people, even if those benefits have rarely come without strings attached. Scholars of medicalization (a concept that will be discussed in greater depth below) have argued that many socially "deviant" behaviors (such as alcoholism and same-sex sexual activity) were considered through the lens of sin and crime prior to the ascent of science and medicine in the late nineteenth century in the West. With the rise of science and medicine, some of these socially deviant behaviors became reconceptualized as symptoms of an illness or disease and the regulation of people engaging in these behaviors or displaying these symptoms moved from the church and the criminal justice system to the hospital and the asylum. According to some scholars, while the medical system is no less regulatory than the criminal justice system, in some cases (but of course not all), the control imposed by the medical system may be less violent than the control imposed by the criminal justice system (Conrad 2007; Foucault 1990, 1994). As Michel Foucault also points out, the identities in-part created by medical and scientific systems (e.g., the identity of the "homosexual") could become focal points of resistance within the system, although they could not escape the orbit of the system itself (Foucault 1990).

It is also the case that some scientists and medical professionals (especially those who were themselves minorities) became advocates, albeit never perfect ones, of the marginalized groups that they "treated." In Europe, for example, Richard von Krafft-Ebing (1840–1902)—considered one of the founders of medical sexology (the classification of different sexual "disorders")—spent his lifetime in correspondence with "sexually deviant" individuals and, probably as a result, eventually began to advocate, in a limited and imperfect capacity, on their behalf by opposing the criminalization of same-sex sexual activity (Oosterhuis 2000). Magnus Hirschfeld (1868–1935), another founder of medical sexology and a sexual minority himself, advocated even more fiercely for sexual and gender minorities in Germany prior to the rise of the Nazis (Mancini 2010). In the United States, the endocrinologist Harry Benjamin (1885–1986), considered one of the founders of "transsexual medicine," was a passionate, albeit imperfect, advocate for "transsexuals" seeking transition-related medical interventions (Ekins 2005). Evelyn Hooker (1907–1996), a psychologist, became an advocate for gays and lesbians, and her research on the mental health of gay men was used to challenge the pathologization of homosexuality by the American Psychiatric Association (Bayer 1987). These are just a few of the individuals who have used their scientific and medical authority to advocate for the rights of marginalized individuals.

In addition, it is important to point out that some marginalized groups and individuals have actively sought scientific and medical support and allyship, and they have worked together with scientists and medical professionals, albeit in hierarchical relationships, to develop medical definitions and treatment protocols. For example, historian Henry Oosterhuis argues that many "sexually deviant" individuals reached out to Richard von Krafft-Ebing to offer him their life stories and their interpretations of their own sexuality and that Krafft-Ebing incorporated many of these interpretations into his own thinking (Oosterhuis 2000). Somewhat similarly, Joanne Meyerowitz argues that transsexual individuals often played an active role (although from a position of subordination) in shaping medical definitions of and approaches to transsexuality (Meyerowitz 2004). It is still the case that some marginalized groups and individuals, including those with "medically unexplained symptoms,"[1] actively seek out the allyship of scientific and medical professionals and seek to define issues as medical problems, although this may be largely because scientific and medical professionals serve as gatekeepers to social, economic, and political support and social legitimacy (Conrad 1992).

And, of course, many marginalized people depend on medical interventions to reduce pain and prolong life. While some people with disabilities do not need medical attention, other people with disabilities, especially people with chronic illnesses like HIV/AIDS, depend on medical interventions to sustain their lives (Wendell 2013). While advancing medical technologies have sometimes led to the reduction or elimination of certain forms of mind/body difference (discussed further below), medical technologies have also enabled new forms of mind/body difference—for example, prematurely born infants who would never have survived in the past are now able to survive as a result of mechanical ventilation, intravenous nutrition, and artificial surfactant (National Research Council. 2007), leading to a new type of being-in-the-world—that of the very premature infant.

AN INTERSECTIONAL FEMINIST CRITIQUE
OF THE HISTORY OF WESTERN BIOMEDICINE

While Western biomedicine has certainly benefited people from marginalized groups, Western biomedicine has also served to reproduce and reinforce sexism, racism, ableism, heterosexism, and colonialism in so many ways that I cannot cover them fully in this chapter. In regards to gender, for example, historically women's bodies have been judged against a (white, heterosexual, able-bodied) male standard and have been deemed lacking and/or excessive, and unhealthy as a result (E. Martin 2001). In addition, women who failed to conform (or overconformed) to racialized feminine stereotypes were diagnosed with various disorders—for example, white-middle class women were diagnosed with hysteria in the late nineteenth and early twentieth centuries for displaying a wide variety of gender-atypical behavior—and non- or overconforming women were forced into compliance with gender norms through medical "treatment" or were confined in medical institutions if they could not be normalized (Briggs 2000).

Similarly, the mind/bodies of people of color were deemed inferior and inherently unhealthy, an ideology that was used to justify slavery and colonial control (Briggs 2002; Levine 1994; Philip 2004; D. E. Roberts 1999; Chakrabarti 2013; Baynton 2013). As in the case of women of all races who resisted gender norms, people of color of all genders who resisted racism were diagnosed with medical illnesses, such as drapetomania in the nineteenth century and schizophrenia in the twentieth century (Duster 2006; Washington 2006; Metzl 2010). Public health officials directly monitored and regulated the behavior of poor people, people of color, and colonized populations (Chakrabarti 2013; Washington 2006; D. E. Roberts 1999). At the same time, people of color in the United States, indigenous people, and colonized populations all over the world have served as "resources" for Western biomedicine—Western biomedicine has developed, in part, by extracting resources (such as drugs, knowledge, cell lines, and genetic material) from indigenous and colonized populations and by using indigenous and colonized populations (especially enslaved African Americans in the United States) as experimental research subjects (Philip 2004; Chakrabarti 2013; Washington 2006). In addition, medical developments have been spurred on by the need to maintain the health of colonial armies and in response to wounds inflicted by imperial and colonial wars (Terry 2009; Chakrabarti 2013).

Sexual and gender minorities were also targeted by Western biomedicine for diagnosis and normalization, although, as noted above, such medical "care" was sometimes preferable to targeting by legal or religious institutions. Throughout the late nineteenth and the first half of the twentieth centuries, much of the medical profession (particularly in the United States) viewed gays and lesbians as physically and/or mentally disordered and used a variety of "treatments," including but not limited to psychotherapy, hormonal injections, and electroshock therapy, in an effort to convert sexually nonconforming subjects to heterosexuality (Terry 1999). While some medical professionals were early allies of trans people, many in the medical profession attempted to impose gender conformity on gender nonconforming people and intersex people (more on this below) (Meyerowitz 2004; Kessler 1998).

Western biomedicine has also served a key role in the oppression of people with disabilities—often viewing people with disabilities as objects of pity in need of a cure and/or institutionalization. Many disability rights activists and disability studies scholars have identified the medical system as one of the primary agents of the oppression of people with disabilities, a point returned to later in this chapter (Wendell 2013; Nielsen 2012).

The history of Western biomedicine includes within it the history of eugenics, which affected poor people, people of color, people with disabilities, and gender and sexual minorities. Eugenics programs included efforts both to encourage the "fittest" members of society to reproduce and to discourage or prevent the "unfit" members of society from reproducing. In the United States, medical professionals participated in eugenics programs by screening immigrants in order to prevent the "unfit" from entering the country and by sterilizing those deemed "unfit" under the legal auspices of eugenic sterilization laws. In the early twentieth century, sterilization programs often targeted a range of poor people, gender and sexual minorities, people of color, and people with disabilities. After the 1950s, these programs often increasingly focused on poor women of color. In Germany under the Nazis, eugenics programs began with sterilization and incarceration and ended with genocide—some of the earliest victims of the Nazis were children and adults with disabilities living in institutional settings inside Germany. Eventually, when the Nazis began to execute Jews and others confined in concentration camps, they used the gassing and crematorium equipment originally developed to execute people with disabilities (Nielsen 2012; Kline 2001; Ordover 2003; Friedlander 1997; Briggs 2002; Lombardo 2010).

While some of biomedicine's worst practices have been eliminated or tempered, sexism, racism, classism, heterosexism, ableism, and colonialism remain very much a part of biomedicine's present. It is to this present that I turn to next.

Medicine as a Stratified and Discriminatory System

Contemporary biomedicine in the United States is stratified both in terms of healthcare workers and in terms of patient access to healthcare. Medicine is organized hierarchically in terms of authority and compensation—with physician administrators and then physicians at the top, nurses and other medical professionals in the middle, and a large pool of "unskilled" healthcare aides at the bottom. In the United States, those at the top are more likely to be white and male and those at the bottom are more likely to be female, of color, and/or immigrants (Lorber and Moore 2002). Within a particular job category (e.g., physician), women and people of color face discrimination and are segregated into lower-status subcategories (e.g., women are more likely to be primary care physicians while men are more likely to be surgeons) (Lorber and Moore 2002; Athanasiou et al. 2016; Laine and Turner 2004; Weaver et al. 2015).

At the same time that the medical profession is stratified, access to medicine is stratified along racial, class, gender, and other lines, and minority patients experience discriminatory treatment at the hands of medical personnel. In the United States, racial and ethnic minorities, low-income people, and members of marginalized groups are less likely to participate in medical trials (although some groups may be overrepresented) and these groups are less likely to have access to healthcare (measured by indicators such as health insurance coverage and delaying or foregoing necessary medical care), although disparities in access have decreased somewhat since the implementation of the Affordable Care Act

(2010) ("Obamacare") (J. Chen et al. 2016; Riley 2012; Derose, Gresenz, and Ringel 2011). As an example, in 2015, 92.5 percent of non-Hispanic whites and non-Hispanic Asians in the United States had health insurance, compared to 88.8 percent of non-Hispanic blacks, 87.4 percent of non-Hispanic Native Hawaiians and Other Pacific Islanders, 78.9 percent of Hispanics and Latinos, and 78.6 percent of non-Hispanic American Indians and Alaskan Natives (U.S. Department of Health and Human Services n.d.).

The situation is more complicated when it comes to gender; as a group, women in the United States are more likely than men to have health insurance and to visit the doctor. This gender disparity is likely the result of a variety of factors, including ideals of masculinity that lead to an underutilization of healthcare services by men, ideals of femininity that place responsibility on women for the health of their spouses and children, the overmedicalization of women's bodies (discussed above and below), and the fact that, in the United States, healthcare for low-income individuals is tied to parental status (U.S. Department of Health and Human Services n.d.; Courtenay 2000; Mahalik, Burns, and Syzdek 2007; Pinkhasov et al. 2010; Noone and Stephens 2008). This gender disparity has positive and negative consequences for both women and men as individuals and as groups; as Will H. Courtenay writes, "The social practices that undermine men's health are often the instruments men use in the structuring and acquisition of power," while the practices, such as care seeking, that lead to higher healthcare utilization by women can also place women under the control of (male) doctors and contribute to the idea "that men's bodies are structurally more efficient than and superior to women's bodies" (Courtenay 2000, 1388–1389, 1395).

In addition to the fact that access to healthcare is stratified by social categories, it is also the case that medical professionals often hold stereotyped views of patients from marginalized social groups, which can negatively impact the healthcare received by these patients. A number of studies have found evidence of racial, gender, and other biases among medical professionals (Balsa and McGuire 2003; Sabin et al. 2009; Fallin-Bennett 2015). Researchers have found that these biases lead to differences in care in a number of areas; for example, studies have found that women who experience myocardial infarction (heart attack) may receive less evidence-based medical care than men (Jneid et al. 2008) and that racial minorities may receive lower-quality pain care than whites (K. O. Anderson, Green, and Payne 2009; Heins et al. 2006; Dickason et al. 2015; Pletcher et al. 2008).

MEDICINE AS PROFIT, NOT PEOPLE, MOTIVATED

One of the primary drivers of medical "innovation" and medicalization (discussed below) has been the desire of medical and pharmaceutical industries to create new patient populations and new conditions to treat in order to increase profits. For example, Ehrenreich and English argue that gynecologists in the early 1900s were motivated in large part by financial interests to pursue the medicalization of childbirth and the criminalization of the mostly female lay healthcare practitioners who had previously provided the majority of birth-related care. According to Ehrenreich and English, the takeover of birth-related care by gynecologists was in many cases detrimental to maternal and fetal health, as gynecologists were more likely than lay healthcare providers to employ risky interventions during labor (Ehrenreich and English 2013).

In the contemporary era, concern over the role of profits in medicine has focused on the pharmaceutical industry. According to critics, pharmaceutical companies have financial incentives to engage in a variety of problematic practices, including encouraging doctors to prescribe drugs for "off-label" use (non-FDA approved use), "ghostwriting" academic articles, manipulating trial results to minimize the appearance of side effects and maximize the appearance of benefits, promoting "academic thought leaders" (medical researchers who are willing to give presentations to other doctors and speak to the media about "disorders" and drug interventions), and, in general, engaging in "disease mongering" and what Gabriel and Goldberg (2014) call "disease inflation." In addition, drug companies have incentives to develop the drugs that they think will be profitable but few incentives to develop needed drugs that are not expected to be profitable (Gabriel and Goldberg 2014; Moynihan and Cassels 2006; Angell 2005; Healy 2004; but see also Pollock 2011). All of these practices are thought to compromise the well-being of patients. Feminist scholars have raised concerns about drug company practices in regards to hormone therapy replacement (Lock 1994), antidepressants (Fullagar 2009), menstrual suppression drugs (Gunson 2010; Mamo and Fosket 2009; Woods 2013), and drugs to treat premenstrual dysphoric disorder (PMDD) (Ussher 2003; Chrisler and Caplan 2002), among others.

The final three critiques of medicine discussed here have mostly (although not exclusively) developed out of the scholarship on medicalization, drawing on the work of Michel Foucault, Peter Conrad, Thomas Szasz, and others. Conrad defines medicalization as follows: "a process by which nonmedical problems become defined and treated as medical problems, usually in terms of illnesses or disorders" (Conrad 1992, 209). Over the past forty years, the scholarship on medicalization has grown in scope and sophistication, and additional terms have been proposed—such as *healthicization, pharmaceuticalization, biocapital, biocitizenship,* and *biomedicalization*—to better capture the ways in which an ever-expanding array of (bio)medical technologies are increasingly used to (self)manage bodies not only to "treat" illness but also to promote "health." In general, scholars of medicalization have argued that more and more aspects of our lives and more and more forms of mind/body diversity have been brought under the purview of medical authority for purposes of social control (see Conrad 1994; A. E. Clarke et al. 2003; Rose 2007; Pollock and Jones 2015).

MEDICINE AS NORMALIZATION

Biomedicine remains an institution of normalization. According to this critique, medical practices are embedded with sexist, racist, heterosexist, classist, and ableist norms, which influence the definition of disease categories and treatment options. These categories and treatments are then brought to bear on nonnormative subjects/patients, either through direct imposition or through a process of self-disciplining.

A number of feminist scholars have examined these processes in regards to women's sexuality and reproduction, arguing that the medical system has tended to regulate these processes according to sexist norms. For example, in an important early work, Margaret Lock examined the medicalization of menopause in the United States. According to Lock, a number of factors contributed to medical understandings of menopause—including worries about heart disease and osteoporosis, economic considerations (primarily the desire of drug companies to sell hormone replacement therapies), and demographic factors, as a growing population of middle-aged women prompted widespread anxiety. In addition, medical approaches were shaped by cultural norms about femininity, including an intense societal antipathy toward female aging and the belief that menopause must be a time of crisis for women, as it involves the loss of reproductive capacities. According to Lock, the medical response to menopause has had serious consequences—as women's bodies have been judged and "treated" according to sexist norms, millions of middle-class white women in the United States have been encouraged to use hormone replacement therapies, with all of the attendant health-related risks (such as increased risk of stroke). Lock writes, "This vision [of menopause], which denies any meaning to aging other than the biological, represents a massive denial of any possible advantages to declining estrogen levels for the aging body; it collapses time and attempts to keep women eternally in the present, dependent and only partially mature" (Lock 1994, 365).

As another example of medicine as a system of normalization, a number of scholars have described how, until very recently, doctors undertook significant medical interventions when an infant was born with "ambiguous" genitalia (genitalia that cannot be easily categorized as male or female, including "micropenises" and "enlarged" clitorises). These doctors believed that parents could not tolerate genital ambiguity and that the possession of "ambiguous" genitalia would lead to mental health disorders in the child as they aged. Accordingly, these doctors selected a male sex/gender for the infant if they felt they could create "normal"-looking male genitalia, or they selected a female sex/gender for the infant if they felt they could create "normal"-looking female genitalia.

According to Suzanne Kessler, these doctors believed that a person's genitals must validate or confirm their gender identity. Kessler writes, "Dichotomized, idealized, and created by surgeons, genitals mean gender [to doctors]. A belief in two genders encourages talk about 'female genitals' and 'male genitals' as homogenous types, regardless of how much variability there is within a category" (Kessler 1998, 132). Thus, the medical response to intersex infants was based on norms about gender, and in turn, the medical management of intersex infants served to reinforce our society's dichotomous gender system, literally through the surgical construction of dichotomous genitalia (see also D. A. Rubin 2017; G. Davis 2015; Reis 2009; Karkazis 2008; Preves 2003; Dreger 2009).

Medicine as Individualizing and Privatizing

A related critique offered by feminist scholars of the medical model is that the medical model locates the cause of all problems within the body/mind while ignoring the influence of social conditions on bodily and mental distress. At the same time, the medical model offers private interventions, such as medicine, surgery, and individual behavior change as a response to all bodily and mental distress.[2] According to scholars, locating the "problem" within the individual and seeking to treat the individual through medication, surgery, or individual behavior change may foreclose efforts to address the broader social and cultural factors (i.e., gender inequality) that may contribute to an individual's bodily and mental distress. Scholars have argued that the medical model meshes well with *neoliberalism* (simply defined, a dominant political and economic ideology that advocates for policies such as privatization, deregulation, free trade, and reduced public spending on social services, among other things). According to this argument, the medical model's focus on placing responsibility for health on the individual citizen as opposed to the state and its focus on individual, monetizable interventions at the expense of social change aligns closely with a neoliberal focus on individual market exchange at the expense of large-scale social welfare projects (on the relationship between medicine and neoliberalism, see, e.g., King 2004; LeBesco 2011; Jarrin 2012; Teghtsoonian 2009; Nygren, Fahlgren, and Johansson 2015).

Dorothy Roberts provides an example of this dynamic in her path-breaking analysis of medical efforts to control the reproduction of black women. Roberts argues that the fertility of black women has been blamed for poverty in black communities, and she describes how medicine has been used to directly control black women's fertility. After World War II, thousands of black women were involuntarily sterilized at the hands of government-paid doctors. Before it was taken off the market in the United States, low-income black women were pressured to use Norplant, a long-lasting form of birth control. According to Roberts, because Norplant must be inserted and removed by a doctor, it decreases a woman's control over her reproductive capacities. Roberts writes, "Underlying these measures are the twin assumptions that the problem of Black poverty can be cured by lowering Black birthrates and that Black women's bodies are an appropriate site for this social experiment" (Roberts 1999, 149; for an examination of the control of Puerto Rican women's sexuality, see Briggs 2002). Similarly, Roberts critiques the approval and marketing of the prescription medication BiDil as a treatment for heart disease in African Americans. According to Roberts, the high rate of heart disease among African Americans is more directly attributable to social factors such as poverty and discrimination, as opposed to genetic factors. Roberts poses the question, "Why not pursue both race-based medicine and social approaches to health inequities, full steam ahead," and answers, "race-specific therapeutics may reduce the public's willingness to change social conditions that impair African Americans' health" (D. E. Roberts 2008, 542). She goes on to argue, "Placing the responsibility for ending health disparities on individual health decisions or on taking race-based medications will weaken the sense of societal obligation to fix systemic inequities" (D. E. Roberts 2008, 542; see also Pollock 2012).

As another example, a number of different scholars have argued that medical (and some public health) approaches to breast cancer promote privatized instead of collective solutions. Audre Lorde was one of the first to articulate this position. In her searing memoir, *The Cancer Journals* (1980), Lorde criticizes exclusively biomedical approaches to breast cancer, calling for collective political action to address the social and environmental causes of breast cancer. She famously asks, "For instance, what would happen if an army of one-breasted women descended on Congress and demanded that the use of carcinogenic fat-stored hormones in beef-feed be outlawed?" (Lorde 1997, 16). Relatedly, based on a qualitative study of women considered "at risk" for breast cancer, Robertson (2000) concludes that the women responded to their anxiety about being "at risk" by engaging in "healthy" lifestyle activities such as low-fat diets, not smoking, controlling their alcohol consumption, practicing stress management strategies, and managing their reproductive options in particular ways, or, if they were not doing these things, they were exhorting themselves to adopt these behavior changes (A. Robertson 2000, 230). According to Robertson, this response

> represents an embodiment of a currently prevailing neo-liberal rationality (Rose, 1990, 1993; Castel, 1991; Burchell, 1993; Greco, 1993; Petersen, 1997) consistent with prevailing discourses on health risk. The argument here is that neo-liberal notions of individual autonomy, the free market and limited government are related, in a mutually producing and sustaining way, to the imperatives of 'self-care'—in the form of self-surveillance and self-regulation—at the heart of prevailing discourses on health risk. . . . It should also, therefore, not be surprising that the women in the present study talked about the man-

agement of breast cancer risk only at an individual level and not at a collective or political level. (A. Robertson 2000, 231)

Finally, Samantha King argues that an initial activist response to breast cancer in the late 1970s and 1980s has been transformed into a privatized philanthropic enterprise. Leading breast cancer advocacy organizations focus on securing donations from individuals, corporations, and foundations in order to "fund the cure" while corporations use breast cancer campaigns to improve their public image and boost their profits. Even the U.S. government has endorsed a privatized approach to breast cancer, as the U.S. Postal Service sold a "breast cancer" stamp that cost one cent more than a regular stamp, promising to donate the extra proceeds to breast cancer research. According to King, "Contemporary discourses, strategies and tools of generosity reflect and produce a remolded view of America as a conflict-free and integrated nation whose survival depends on personal acts of philanthropy mediated through—and within—consumer culture. By according responsibility for the health and welfare of individuals to personal generosity, we simultaneously deploy a constricted understanding of the economic, political, social and cultural forces that converge to shape problems of health and welfare" (King 2004, 489; see also Klawiter 2008).[3]

Eugenics has also reemerged within Western biomedicine in a neoliberal guise. Medical technologies like preimplantation genetic diagnosis (PGD) and prenatal testing have given potential parents the option to select against bearing children with specific genetic differences (e.g., children with Down syndrome). Some bioethicists have applauded this development, calling it the "new eugenics" because the state is not dictating what kinds of people will be brought into the world; instead, individual parents will be able to make choices in order to enhance human health and human capacities (Savulescu 2001; Savulescu and Kahane 2009). However, as many scholars have pointed out, the "new eugenics" is likely to produce the same kinds of discriminatory decisions that were produced by the "old" eugenics, even if those decisions are now being made by individuals rather than the state. The collective result of individuals making decisions within systems of inequality may lead to the elimination of certain types of disabilities—or more poignantly—certain types of people from the world (Sparrow 2011; Daar 2017). For example, in her analysis of genetic testing, Rayna Rapp argues that genetic testing requires women to make individual choices about whether to continue a pregnancy after learning of a genetic "anomaly." According to Rapp, this means that our society avoids engaging in a conversation about "who should be allowed entry into the human community." She writes, "Ending a pregnancy . . . because of a particular diagnosed disability forces each woman to act as a moral philosopher of the limits, adjudicating the standards guarding entry into the human community for which she serves as normalizing gatekeeper" (Rapp 2004, 131). As disability studies scholars have argued, genetic testing followed by abortion is an individual solution (the abortion of the "disabled" fetus) that allows our society to avoid addressing social problems, including the stigma attached to disability, the lack of resources available for parenting a child with a disability, and social obstacles blocking people with disabilities from participating fully in communal life (Wendell 2013; Hubbard 2013; Saxton 2013).[4]

However, feminist scholars have also argued that even politically informed alternatives to biomedicine can be implicated in the system of neoliberal capitalism. For example, in *Seizing the Means of Reproduction*, Michelle Murphy argues that while the alternative do-it-yourself health practices developed by radical feminists in California in the 1970s and 1980s were intended to operate outside of the commoditized system of mainstream medicine, they shared with neoliberal medical approaches an emphasis on self-monitoring and individual responsibility for one's own body and health. In addition, some of the innovative technologies developed by feminist health care activists were eventually coopted and marketed for profit (Murphy 2012).

Overall, it is indisputable that a biomedical framework encourages us to understand and respond to bodily and mental distress in a particular way. In summarizing the view that medical discourses and practices may limit the way we address problems, Jana Sawicki echoes Dorothy Roberts, writing, "There may be better solutions; and there may be better ways of defining the problems. There is the danger that medical solutions will become the only ones and that other ways of defining [problems] will be eclipsed" (Sawicki 1991, 85). While I certainly share the concern expressed by Roberts and Sawicki, I do ultimately argue for combining biomedical approaches with collective solutions to social problems. Many of the critiques of biomedicine as an (inappropriately) individualized approach seem to view the relationship between the social and the individual as unidirectional: societal forces become embodied/minded, but changes in the body/mind do not seem to produce changes in social structures. Drawing from a feminist science studies perspective, I argue, instead, that biomedical interventions that change an individual's body/mind do have the potential to produce social change; as a hypothetical example, consider the case of a woman who is experiencing severe anxiety in part as a result of sexual harassment on the job, who takes an antianxiety medication that enables her to pursue a sexual harassment case against her employer without experiencing a panic attack. Of course, in most cases, as I argued in the Introduction, individual biomedical interventions serve to shore up social systems of oppression by replicating problematic norms, mitigating the worst of the system's negative effects, and draining away discontent that might otherwise have been mobilized to support more radical political projects. Still, as I also argued in the Introduction, feminists must also acknowledge that social change can be difficult and slow. My position is that in some cases, people should not be asked to forgo individual solutions to pain while waiting for systemic changes. In addition, in some cases, systemic injustice may have already caused significant harms that will not be soothed by changing the system to prevent future harms; in a subset of these cases, individual solutions may bring some comfort. I advocate for pursuing collective transformation while allowing for individual interventions, with the recognition that those individual interventions may make collective transformation more difficult to achieve.

MEDICINE AS ALIENATING AND DISPLACING

Another critique of medicine developed by feminist scholars is that medicine increases our reliance on medical experts and undermines our privileged relationship to our own bodies, while displacing alternative ways of understanding mind/body distress. Feminist disability studies scholar Susan Wendell argues that medicine can lead to alienation from our bodies and to epistemic invalidation, or the denial of our ability to produce and transmit knowledge about our own bodies. To start, medicine requires patients to use the language of medicine to describe themselves and their bodies, rather than phenomenological descriptions, or descriptions deriving from personal embodied experience (I provide an example below). In addition, according to Wendell, the knowledge that we have about our own bodies (e.g., as ailing) is not accepted as valid by society unless we receive a diagnosis from a medical professional. Thus, medical professionals are allowed to adjudicate who is deserving of social support, and people without a medical diagnosis may be abandoned by family, friends, and social institutions. Based on this analysis, Wendell argues very strongly that social need should not be determined by medical classifications, a position that I adopt here and expand on later (Wendell 2013).

In her analysis of menstruation, menopause, and childbirth, Emily Martin echoes similar themes. Martin argues that during childbirth, medical professionals often view women as simply containers for laboring uteri. According to Martin, this encourages women to view themselves as separate from the process of labor, and, in fact, the women she interviewed largely described menstruation, menopause, and labor contractions as separate from the self. In her study, when asked to explain menstruation to a young girl, middle-class women also used medical and scientific language to describe their experiences with menstruation (describing, for example, eggs moving from the ovaries through the fallopian tubes to the uterus and then passing out of the body as blood if not fertilized) (E. Martin 2001). In contrast, many of the working-class women in her study used phenomenological language to describe their experiences with menstruation, for example, when asked to explain menstruation to a young girl, one woman said, "I would tell her that her menstrual is like one of the worst nightmares. . . . With it comes displeasure because one, your period makes me sick because the blood, it ain't got the best odor in the world and I would tell her to check with the pharmacist for the best thing to use. . . . But the Kotex is very uncomfortable. It is like a big bulk. And you feel it close to you and it is an icky feeling" (E. Martin 2001, 108–109).

Iris Marion Young also argues that childbirth in a medical context can lead to epistemic invalidation. According to Young, women are not considered valuable sources of information about the status of the fetus. Rather, doctors rely on instruments, such as sonograms, to gain knowledge "directly" about the fetus. Thus, through the use of instruments, the physician devalues the privileged relation the woman has to the fetus and to her body (I. M. Young 2005).

In addition to displacing individual phenomenological understandings of the mind/body, scholars have argued that the institution of Western biomedicine has intentionally and unintentionally devalued and displaced non-Western and indigenous values, knowledge systems, and practices of healing. For example, as discussed in greater depth in Chapter 3, trans studies scholars have argued that Western biomedical approaches to trans experience can render "invisible the cultural diversity of gender expressions and identities worldwide" and can impose "an exclusive framework of conceiving gender diversity" on non-Western societies (Suess, Espineira, and Walters 2014, 74–75; see also Najmabadi 2008, 2013; Namaste 2011; Stryker 2012).

Taken as a whole, these critiques of medicine and medical technologies paint a damning picture of the role of medicine in the lives of women, people of color, sexual and gender minorities, and people with disabilities. And yet, many scholars and activists have retained a belief in the value of biomedical approaches. These scholars and activists have adopted at least two general strategies to defend or recuperate medicine from feminist critiques: celebrating individual agency in the use of medical technologies and/or arguing that yes, medicine can be abused to enforce social norms but that it also can relieve suffering and thus we must simply restrict medicine to cases of "true" illness. Here I will briefly summarize these responses and where I think they fail and where they offer valuable insight.

Celebrating Agency

This position tends to argue that women (and others) can freely choose whether to use a particular medical intervention, and as such, it is a feminist obligation to respect or even celebrate a women's use of a medical intervention as an expression of her agency and autonomy. This position is one that few (if any) feminist activists or scholars have taken themselves, at least in its stark form. However, feminist scholars have found that some of the women who chose "suspect" medical interventions do see themselves as exercising agency. For example, from her interviews with female cosmetic surgery patients in the Netherlands, Kathy Davis found that many of the women saw their cosmetic surgeries as empowering and positive self-made choices (K. Davis 1994; see also Pitts-Taylor 2007). Occasionally, this position is reflected in pop/activist feminist writing on the issue. For example, in an article for *New Internationalist* magazine, self-identified feminist blogger Danielle Leigh writes, "As the term 'liberation' is so subjective, if someone believes that their surgery has liberated them then we must surely take their word for it. When we begin to challenge a person's ability to decide for themselves whether or not their surgery has had a positive impact on their lives, we tread on very dangerous ground" (Leigh and Logeais 2014, n.p.). Yet, hopefully it is clear from what I have already said that this position is not a wholly adequate response to feminist, queer, antiracist, and crip critiques of medicine, as these critiques have demonstrated that individual decisions to use a particular medical intervention are produced within and may serve to perpetuate a social context in which some types of body/minds are valued and others are devalued. We do not have to believe that people are victims of false consciousness to recognize that individual desires are influenced by social norms about what counts as a healthy (equated with good) mind/body. We can certainly recognize the agency of people making choices within structures of constraint, but we cannot ignore the fact that some choices, typically choices to use medical interventions in the service of normalization, are rewarded by society, while other choices, typically choices to refuse medical intervention or to use medical interventions to resist normalization, are punished. In addition, as I discussed before, when individuals exercise agency and make choices within oppressive systems, the collective result of those decisions can be harmful to marginalized individuals and groups. Thus, any straightforward celebration of agency in this context is not tenable.

A modified version of this position, one endorsed by many feminist scholars and activists and one that I use to a certain extent here, views decisions such as the decision to undergo cosmetic surgery as potentially rational responses to current conditions. In regards to cosmetic surgery, for example, Rosemary Gillespie writes, "Cosmetic surgery may serve to reinforce limited and restrictive models of femininity. Collusion with these processes, it is suggested, may be rational for some women at the individual level as they seek to increase their social power in a society where women are judged by their appearance more than men. At the social level, however, such action can be seen to go against women's collective interests and perpetuate wider social inequalities" (Gillespie 1997, 69). This modified position, however, is less a defense of medicine than it is a way of understanding the actions of those who undertake medical interventions, and it is possible to hold this position and argue that even though medical interventions may be "rational" for individual patients, because they have a negative effect at the societal level, these interventions should still be opposed.

Taking the discussion of agency in a different direction, some scholars and activists have argued that it is possible for individuals to appropriate medical interventions for their own purposes and use these interventions to subvert dominant norms. For example, in *Testo Junkie: Sex, Drugs, and Biopolitics in the Pharmacopornographic Era*, Paul B. Preciado describes taking black-market testosterone gel for a year as "an auto-experimental form of do-it-yourself bioterrorism of gender" (Preciado 2013, 389). Preciado writes, "I'm not taking testosterone to change myself into a man or as a physical strategy of transsexualism; I take it to foil what society wanted to make of me, so that I can write, fuck, feel a form of pleasure that is postpornographic, add a molecular prostheses to my low-tech transgender identity composed of dildos, texts, and moving images" (Preciado 2013, 16).

As another example, Kathryn Pauly Morgan argues that feminists could appropriate cosmetic surgery to make themselves look "ugly" as a way of subverting patriarchal beauty norms (Morgan 1991), and Victoria Pitts-Taylor argues that performance artist Orlan has, in a sense, done exactly this by undertaking plastic surgeries that radically subvert normative beauty standards (Pitts-Taylor 2007, 82–84). In a somewhat similar vein, Cressida J. Heyes argues that while medical practices (such as dieting, cosmetic surgery, and "sex-reassignment surgery") are disciplinary practices, these practices are also self-care practices and can produce capacities such as self-reflection and self-control. According to Heyes, while these new capacities are usually placed in the service of normalization, they could also be used to open up unanticipated possibilities (Heyes 2007).

Yet, as most of these activists and scholars note, it is difficult to use mainstream medical interventions in a radically subversive matter. As noted above, practices that seem to be subversive may actually reinforce hierarchies (as in the case of neoprimitivist body modification undertaken by queer white subjects referenced in the Introduction). In addition, the medical system itself often works hard to ensure that medical interventions are used to promote normalization. For example, Dean Spade writes of his desire to see a variety of practices, including surgery and hormones, used to "promote sex reassignment, gender alteration, temporary gender adventure, and the mutilation of gender categories," but points out that the medical establishment often only grants access to surgery and hormones when the patient promises to use them in the service of gender normativity (Spade 2003, 21). It seems clear that, in most cases, medical interventions are employed by a majority of their users to pursue normalization and only a small percentage of users employ these interventions for nonnormative ends.

RESTRICT THE DEFINITION OF ILLNESS

A second common response to feminist critiques of medicine has been to argue that many conditions have been improperly medicalized and subjected to intervention but that medicine should not be abandoned altogether; rather, we should more carefully restrict the use of medicine to cases of "true" illness. This response hinges on our ability to separate "true" illness/pathology from "normal" bodily and mental variation. There is a large body of literature in the philosophy of medicine on the definition of illness categories, which I summarize here. Some thinkers have attempted to draw the line between illness and health based on so-called objective criteria (sometimes called "naturalistic" approaches). For example, modifying earlier work by Christopher Boorse, bioethicist Norman Daniels argues that, in a just society, medical care for citizens should be covered when it is designed to restore "species-typical functioning" (Daniels 2000, 2001, 2007). The definition of species-typical functioning depends both on evolutionary design and statistical averages: according to this theory, we can determine what is the evolutionarily evolved function of bodily parts and processes (e.g., we can determine that the heart evolved to pump blood through the body), and we can determine what is the statistically typical level of functioning of bodily parts and processes (e.g., we can determine what is the statistically average ability of hearts to pump blood). Disability or disease, then, is any functioning that falls below the species-typical level (see Kingma 2007; Krag 2014; Guerrero 2010). According to Daniels, "The line between disease and disability and normal functioning is thus drawn in the relatively objective and nonevaluative context provided by the biomedical sciences, broadly construed" (Daniels 2000, 315). However, as many critics have pointed out, the definition of "species-typical functioning" is chock full with values, and this definition requires equating statistical averages with "normality" (Kingma 2007; Krag 2014; Guerrero 2010). More generally, as Susan Wendell points out, any definition of illness or disability that references what is "normal" or "typical" for a person requires value judgments (Wendell 2013).

Other scholars do not rely on a so-called naturalist definition of disease or disability, acknowledging the role that social and cultural factors play in our definitions of health and illness, but still affirm that we must draw a normative line between genuine and nongenuine medical conditions in order to prevent the improper medicalization of benign human variation ("normative" approaches). For example, Robert Sparrow argues that "notions of the normal are socially constructed and both express and reflect value judgments" (Sparrow 2013b, 191) and that our current understanding of what is normal must be expanded to include a greater amount of bodily and mental variation; however, he also argues that it is strategically necessary to hold onto some conception of what is normal in order to prevent the overuse of medical technologies in cases where the intent is to make someone better than normal (enhancement). To offer my own example, his reasoning suggests that we must have some understanding that height varies within a normal range; otherwise, we will be tempted (and/or obligated) to find out what is the most advantageous height in our society and then use medical interventions to make everyone reach exactly that height. Sparrow argues that holding onto a "queerer" conception of what is normal will actually protect some diversity as it will prevent the use of medical interventions to eliminate all of the forms of bodily and mental variation that we consider normal (Sparrow 2011, 2013b). While I am sympathetic to some of Sparrow's points, as he acknowledges, even "any new, more inclusive, conception of the normal will still exclude some forms of embodiment, which may then eventually be eliminated from societies in which [preimplantation genetic diagnosis] is available" (Sparrow 2013b, 192). In a later work, Sparrow suggests that intersex conditions may fall outside the realm of the normal (Sparrow 2013a), thus demonstrating that even his "queer" definition of normal could lead to the elimination of nonnormative subjects (see Gupta and Freeman 2013).

Given that attempts to categorically separate illness from health either serve to naturalize and essentialize socially constructed categories and/or almost inevitably place some people and conditions on the "wrong" side of the line (either deeming people sick who do not see themselves as disordered or withholding a medical label from those who seek a diagnosis), in this book, I take the position that it is neither necessary nor helpful to define illness categorically. In other words, I argue that it is ultimately counterproductive to define specific conditions as diseases, such that all of the people with a condition defined as a disease are considered ill and worthy of medical intervention and all of the people without a condition defined as a disease are considered healthy and unworthy of medical intervention. Rather, I suggest that it is more helpful to decide the merits of medical intervention based not on whether someone falls into a specific disease/disorder category but based on whether a medical intervention is critical for a person to flourish, based an individual's specific circumstances, with reference to her community and to the broader society. This is an argument that I develop throughout the three case studies and discuss more systematically in the concluding chapter.

SUMMING IT UP

Like other mainstream institutions in a white, capitalist, imperialist patriarchy, the medical system is stratified, both in terms of its workers and in terms of the services it provides to patients. It has served as a system of control and normalization (both of majority and minority populations and of internally and externally colonized populations), has risked the well-being of patients in the interests of profit, and has offered privatized, individualized solutions to social problems. It has also served to invalidate other, potentially valuable, ways of understanding the mind/body, including non-Western approaches to health and healing.

I have argued in this chapter that while we can certainly acknowledge and understand the agency of patients in choosing to undergo particular medical interventions, we must also acknowledge that people might make choices that ultimately have negative consequences for others and for society at large and that all choices take place within a context where conformity to mind/body norms is rewarded and deviance from mind/body norms is punished. I have also argued that while it may be helpful to think carefully about our definitions of illness and health, and that such an undertaking may prevent us from medicalizing certain bodily and mental states unnecessarily, it is not possible to define our way out of moral and political ambiguity and complexity. As I have indicated above, improving our categorical definitions of disease may help prevent abuses but cannot satisfactorily determine who should receive a medical intervention and who should not.

With this background in place, I now turn to a detailed analysis of three case studies: transition-related care, sexuopharmaceuticals, and weight-loss interventions. Each case demonstrates the enormous complexity of the ethical and political issues involved in medical interventions that touch on social categories such as race, class, gender, sexuality, and/or ability.

CHAPTER 3

Theorizing from Transition-Related Care

ANALYTICAL TOOLS FOR COMPLEXITY

In this chapter, I examine the ethics and politics of transition-related care (including but not limited to what is often referred to as "sex-confirmation" or "sex-reassignment" surgery) for transgender individuals who seek to use medical interventions to alter their mind/bodies in sex/gender-relevant ways. Transition-related care has been the focus of a long history of trans activism and has been the subject of a significant body of feminist, queer, and trans scholarship. Both trans-affirming and trans-exclusionary activists and scholars have critiqued the medical establishment for employing transition-related care in the service of gender normalization—in other words, according to these critiques, the ideology and practice of transition-related care has reflected and reinforced the idea that gender identity is an innate property of the body/mind, gender identity is binary (masculine or feminine), and gender identity must match a specific form of sexed embodiment (male or female, respectively).

Additionally, some activist and scholars, of all stripes, have critiqued trans people who seek transition-related care for participating in a system of gender normalization. This critique has been offered in a virulent fashion by some trans-exclusionary feminist activists and scholars (more on this later). Given this history of transphobia in U.S. feminist activism and scholarship, I need to affirm here my unequivocal conviction that trans individuals should have access to high-quality and affirming transition-related care. I am certain that this care is necessary for many trans people to build livable lives.

The purpose of this chapter, then, is not to debate whether trans people should have access to transition-related care but rather to tease out the different social and political implications of this care as it is currently conceptualized and delivered and to explore different options for how this care could be conceptualized and delivered in ways that are less sexist, heterosexist, classist, racist, and ableist. It is my contention that trans-affirming activists and scholars who have worked on the issue of transition-related care have developed highly nuanced theoretical apparatuses that are capable of holding together a critique of the normalizing power of medicine along with an affirmation of the power of medical technologies to make some lives more livable and, in some cases, to promote flourishing.

Before turning to a discussion of transition-related care generally, I introduce a specific case that reveals some of the complicated issues involved in transition-related care in a concrete manner. The case I introduce is that of a transwoman in Florida who performed unlicensed silicone injections and who was convicted of manslaughter in 2017 after one of her clients died. Her story, and the story of her clients, highlights the current failures of the medical system to meet the needs of transgender people in an affirming way and also reveals the complicated relationship between sex/gender-related medical interventions and gender normalization.

With this concrete case as a basis, I move to a more general discussion of transition-related care and its history, along with a history of feminist, queer, and trans approaches to transition-related care. I then turn to outlining critiques of transition-related care as it is currently delivered before turning to a discussion of how this care might be reconceptualized and reformed. I conclude by highlighting the lessons that can be learned from trans-affirming approaches to medicine.

THEORIZING FROM REAL LIVES: ILLEGAL SILICONE INJECTIONS

As part of their transition, some transwomen seek implants and/or injections in order to augment different parts of their bodies. Because these procedures may not be covered by health insurance, and because they can be extremely expensive when performed by a licensed medical provider, some transwomen turn to unlicensed practitioners, often other transwomen, for injections of liquid silicone. Even if the injected silicone is medical grade, there are significant risks involved, and unlicensed practitioners may use nonmedical grade silicone or other fillers, which can increase the risk of complications (Styperek et al. 2013).[1]

In 2017, the story of one unlicensed practitioner, Oneal Ron Morris, made national news after she plead guilty to "manslaughter" following the death of one of her clients. Morris, a transwoman, had injected herself with silicone and had been selling silicone injections to others for years in South Florida. She first made the news in 2011 when she was sentenced to a year in jail for practicing medicine without a license after one of her clients suffered severe complications. Allegedly, Morris had used a mixture of cement, glue, mineral oil, and tire sealant in her injections (G. Nelson 2011a). After the news of Morris's first arrest spread, more former clients came forward, alleging wrongdoing. One of these clients was Rajee Narinesingh, another transwoman, who allegedly received facial injections from Morris that contained different fillers, including cement. Narinesingh told reporters that she was desperate to have plastic surgery and heard about Morris through "word of mouth" in the transgender community. Explaining her reasons for going to Morris, Narinesingh said, "It becomes so dire that you want to match your outside with your inside that you're willing to roll the dice and take your chances" (G. Nelson 2011b). She also told reporters that she trusted Morris because "there was a sisterhood of trust. She was part of the transgender community herself" (Anderson-Minshall 2012).

Shatarka Nuby was another former client who came forward, writing to the Florida State Health Department from a Florida prison. A few months after contacting the health department, she died of respiratory failure due to "massive silicone migration." Morris was charged with Nuby's death in 2012 and pleaded no contest to the charge of manslaughter in 2017. Morris was sentenced to ten years in prison and five years of probation and is reportedly serving her prison sentence in a men's prison (Mettler 2017; Mettler and *Washington Post* 2017).[2]

The case of Morris, Nuby, Narinesingh, and Morris's other clients brings to light a number of complicated issues about transition-related medical interventions. For decades, many trans people seeking medical interventions have been forced to take significant risks, turning to self-treatment, unlicensed practitioners, and/or unproven or dangerous procedures because they cannot access professional medical care—because they cannot afford it, because there are no providers in their area, and/or because they have been turned away by licensed providers for various reasons. Joanne Meyerowitz details some of this history in *How Sex Changed: A History of Transsexuality in the United States* (2004). This history, and the recent example of Morris and her clients, demonstrates how critical access to medical intervention is for some trans people—some trans people are willing to risk death in order to make their body/minds more livable. At the same time, an intersectional analysis is illuminating here as the racial and class aspects of this case cannot be ignored—Morris, Nuby, Narinesingh, and presumably many of Morris's other clients were poor and/or of color and thus more vulnerable to victimization.

In addition to highlighting a long history of exploitation and danger, particularly of poor transwomen of color, the case also highlights a history of trans innovation and self-reliance. Denied professional medical care, trans individuals and communities have developed lay healthcare practices such as the self-administration of hormone therapies and silicone injections. Although these lay healthcare practices can be risky and, in some cases, deadly, they also allow trans people to access medical interventions without needing the approval of traditional medical gatekeepers. Thus, these lay health practices suggest that we might be able to improve the delivery of transition-related care by expanding the orbit of people who can legally deliver these interventions beyond traditional medical professionals.

At the same time, the Morris case raises thorny questions about gender normalization. While some of Morris's clients were transwomen, others were, reportedly, ciswomen and cismen (apparently including Nuby). Some of the press reports do not even mention that Morris served trans clients (e.g., Morrill 2017). At the same time, there have been a number of news stories about ciswomen seeking unlicensed silicone injections. These articles suggest that women are risking life and limb to attain normative standards of feminine beauty. For example, one reporter writes, "This scenario highlights the trick bag many American women find themselves stuck in when they try to meet all the unrealistic expectations of society—run a household, work a full time job, and look like a video girl—all at the same time" (W. L. Cooper 2015, n.p.). Some news stories connect the two phenomena, arguing that trans communities were the first to embrace unlicensed injections and that ciswomen followed suit. For example, the same reporter writes, "What I discovered . . . was that although underground butt injections may have started on the fringes—among the trans community, sex workers, and strippers—women from all walks of life are now willing to gamble with their health in the hope of getting a butt like J. Lo or Nicki Minaj" (W. L. Cooper 2015, n.p.). If trans and ciswomen are using the same procedures—illegal silicone injections—in pursuit of the same goal—"feminine-looking" buttocks— then do these types of interventions merely serve to reinforce problematic appearance-related gender norms? And, in fact, if these interventions are being developed by transwomen and then adopted by ciswomen, are transwomen innovators in the field of gender normalization?

Yet, the picture is even more complicated than is suggested by these questions. Appearance-related gender norms do not exist apart from racial and class norms. Some reporters suggest that (poor) women of color were the first to embrace unlicensed silicone injections and that white and wealthy women followed in their footsteps. For example, one article states, "Very big buttocks have been popular in hip-hop videos for years. But Dionne Stephens, who studies race, gender and sexuality in hip-hop culture at Florida International University, said celebrities such as Jennifer Lopez, Beyonce and Kim Kardashian are popularizing the look among an increasing number of women of all races and ethnicities" (Mohr 2013, n.p.). Again, the language here is of contagion—in some articles, the transfer suggested is from transwomen to ciswomen; in others, the transfer is from women of color to white women. The reporters writing about the Morris case assume that Morris looks monstrous as a result of her "botched" procedures. For example, a reporter for the *Washington Post* writes, "For years in Florida, Morris's name—and posterior—have been widely reported and eventually made national headlines when photos of [her] surfaced. She reportedly used the same cut-rate cosmetic methods that sickened or killed others to inject her own hips and buttocks, leaving them abnormally large and misshapen" (Mettler 2017, n.p.).[3] While I do not know how Morris herself feels about the appearance of her hips and buttocks, what can be said is that many people, trans and cis, sought Morris out and paid her to inject their own buttocks. This suggests that they did not find her appearance repellent, or they would not have paid for her services; in some way, her "abnormally large and misshapen buttocks" were quite literally objects of desire. I suspect that at least some of the media outrage about the Morris case was the result of white, middle-class abhorrence for the gender practices of poor women of color, evidenced by the focus of reporters on the photos of Morris and on the sensational details of the case, such as Morris's use of "Fix-a-Flat" sealant. The media coverage of Morris brings to mind Uma Narayan's critique of Western commentary on the phenomenon of dowry-murders in India; Western commentators tended to focus on what they saw as the grisly and exotic aspects of dowry-murders—the fact that women were being burned to death—rather than seeing burning as a practical and efficient method of murder in households that use pressurized kerosene stoves for cooking (Narayan 2013, 102). The racial aspects of the Morris case raise the question, does it matter which gender norms transwomen are seeking to meet? Are transition-related medical interventions more, less, or equally techniques of normalization if they are used to conform to nonhegemonic appearance-related gender norms?

Finally, as has already been suggested, the Morris case highlights the fact that both transition-related care *and* the sex/gender-related medical procedures undertaken by ciswomen are sensationalized by the media. As noted above, the media coverage of Morris focused on Morris's appearance and the fact that she may have used tire sealant (specifically "Fix-a-Flat" tire sealant) in her injections. The media gave Morris a variety of nicknames, including the "Toxic Tush doctor" and the "Fix-a-Flat" doctor, while also noting that her patients called her "Dutchess" (Mettler 2017; Conti 2017). The case received further notoriety in 2012 when Morris's alleged assistant, a man named Corey Eubank, went on a Spanish-language talk show and was attacked by one of Morris's alleged victims, Shaquanda Brown. Additional attention was brought to the case in 2016, when Rajee Narinesingh (the transwoman who received facial injections from Morris) appeared on *Botched*, an E! television show that follows doctors as they "remedy extreme plastic surgeries gone wrong" (Escobar 2016). The sensationalized coverage of the case reflects a longstanding public fascination with the details of transition-related medical procedures (Serano 2007) and with the bodies of women of color (Gilman 1985). And yet, even the news articles that focus on ciswomen seeking unlicensed silicone injections adopt a sensationalized tone. One article describes women who have received liquid silicone injections as carrying around a "ticking time bomb" (L. Lucas 2015). Another article describes the problem as follows: "The rising demand for the derriere extraordinaire has driven desperate people to put their lives in the hands of anyone wielding a needle—often unaware of the toxic concoction inside" (Crocker and Dickson 2012, n.p.).

In general, the articles present women as reckless and willing to do anything in order to look like their favorite celebrities. One article begins, "Women across the U.S. are risking their lives for illegal procedures to make their buttocks bigger. . . . Some want to fill out a bikini or a pair of jeans. Others believe a bigger bottom will bring them work as music video models or adult entertainers. Whatever the reason, they are seeking cheaper alternatives to plastic surgery—sometimes with deadly or disfiguring results" (Mohr 2013, n.p.). These analyses suggest that women are foolish, unwitting dupes of feminine beauty standards and/or ignorant about the real risks of unlicensed procedures. In general, the sensationalized and paternalistic coverage of trans- and ciswomen seeking unlicensed injections serves to further complicate the task of theorizing transition-related medical interventions. Discussions, such as the one undertaken in this chapter, can feed into the public's fascination with transition-related medical interventions at the expense of seeing trans people as people. The focus on transition-related medical interventions serves to equate transgender experience with the desire to obtain a particular form of sexed embodiment, rather than seeing transgender experience as involving a complex interplay between embodiment, individual life history, interpersonal relationships, communities, and broader social, cultural, political, and economic factors.

The Morris case, then, highlights both the need for increasing access to high-quality transition-related care but also the complex enmeshment of transition-related care in regimes of gender and racial normalization. The case also highlights the potential pitfalls of talking about transition-related medical interventions in an isolated fashion; as such, discussions can serve to equate trans experience with medical intervention. With these issues in mind, I turn to a more generalized discussion of transition-related care, while attempting to not lose sight of particularity in the effort to produce some generally applicable conclusions.

DEFINING TRANS AND TRANSITION-RELATED CARE

In contemporary U.S. society, "trans" is often used as an umbrella term for a variety of gender-nonconforming experiences. Drawing on language and concepts developed primarily by medical professionals like John Money who worked with trans and intersex individuals in the 1950s and 1960s (Meyerowitz 2008; D. A. Rubin 2012), trans has often been represented in the United States as follows: a person's "gender identity" (or the gender they feel themselves to be) is felt to be in conflict with their "sex" (or the sexually dimorphic characteristics of their body)—summarized by the (problematic) phrase "sex is between our legs and gender identity is between our ears" (for examples, see Heldman 2009; Tate 2017). In this particular trans discourse, medical interventions are presented as a way to bring the sex of the body in line with the gender identity of the mind.

Of course, trans, feminist, and queer scholars, activists, and community members have long argued that the reality is more complex than what is suggested by the phrase "gender is between our ears and sex is between our legs" (e.g., Salamon 2010; Prosser 1998; Butler 1993; Stryker 2009). The sex/gender distinction itself has been critiqued for its separation of biology and body ("sex") from culture and mind ("gender") (Butler 1993; Fausto-Sterling 2005). In a still "mass-market" formulation that abandons the language of sex altogether, the National Center for Transgender Equality (NCTE) uses the term "transgender" to refer to people "whose gender identity is different from the gender they were thought to be at birth," thus emphasizing that "gender" assignment at birth is a social process (National Center for Transgender Equality 2016). NCTE goes on to describe transitioning as follows: "Transitioning is the time period during which a person begins to live according to their gender identity, rather than the gender they were thought to be at birth. While not all transgender people transition, a great many do at some point in their lives. Gender transition looks different for every person . . . some people undergo hormone therapy or other medical procedures to change their physical characteristics and make their body better reflect the gender they know themselves to be." Although this description of gender transitioning is accessible, inclusive, and politically practical (yay!), it still suggests that gender is a thing that is knowable prior to transition (I can know myself to be a particular gender) and that the body can be acted on to simply *reflect* one's already known (preexisting) gender identity. This formulation thus essentializes, to an extent, gender identity and ignores the ways in which hormone therapy and other medical procedures act on both the body and mind and the ways in which gender identity may transform and develop during a process of gender transitioning.

Writing for a different audience and with different political goals, Susan Stryker uses the term "transgender" to refer to people "who move away from their birth-assigned gender because they feel strongly that they properly belong to another gender in which it would be better for them to live; others want to strike out toward some new location, some space not yet clearly defined or concretely occupied; still others simply feel the need to get away from the conventional expectations bound up with the gender that was initially put upon them. In any case, it is *the movement across a socially imposed boundary away from an unchosen starting place*—rather than any particular destination or mode of transition" (Stryker 2009, 1).

For the purposes of this chapter, I want to combine Stryker's formulation of transgender with the compound concepts "sex/gender" and "mind/body." The compound "sex/gender" has been developed by scholars in the field of feminist science studies to indicate that there is not a clear-cut distinction between "sex" and "gender" or the "biological" and the "social." The "biology" of "sex" is always shaped by and read through the "sociocultural" lens of "gender," and at the same time, cultural views of gender are shaped by the agency of biological matter, in a constant, dynamic, and iterative process of co-constitution (Dussauge and Kaiser 2012; Barad 2007; Kirby 1997; E. A. Wilson 2004). Similarly, the compound "mind/body" is meant to indicate that the mind is embodied and the body is "mindful" and that both are socially embedded (E. A. Wilson 2015; Scheper-Hughes and Lock 1987). Combining Stryker's formulation with the concepts of sex/gender and mind/body, here I conceptualize transgender most broadly as a disidentification with one's sex/gender of assignment. I conceptualize the desire for transition-related medical care more specifically as a desire to use medical interventions to alter some sexed/gendered aspects of the mind/body, in order to move away from one's sex/gender of assignment, either toward a different socially recognized sex/gender category or toward some "new location," with the recognition that for many trans-identified people, including, perhaps, the clients who sought out Morris's services, transition-related medical care can promote flourishing and may even be life-saving, as pretransition minds/bodies may be distressing or even unlivable. Transition-related medical interventions then are not different from the sex/gender-relevant medical interventions undertaken by cisgender people in terms of their content (indeed, as we saw in the case of Morris, many of the procedures are the same), but rather in their aim—a move away from, rather than toward, one's sex/gender of assignment and in the fact that they involve, in Stryker's terms, movement across a socially imposed boundary.[4] Transition-related medical interventions are thus always, to a certain extent, norm transgressing; however, as we will see, some types of transitions have achieved a seminormative status while others remain extremely marginalized.

TRANSITION-RELATED CARE: SCOPE AND HISTORY

Although the general public may equate "transition-related care" with "genital surgery," in fact, the scope of transition-related care can be much broader than genital surgery or, for many trans people, may not include genital surgery at all. Transition-related care may include hair removal or hair reconstruction/transplantation, hormone therapy (typically testosterone for transmasculine people and testosterone blockers plus estrogen for transfeminine people), "top surgeries" (typically breast removal for transmasculine people and breast augmentation for transfeminine people), "bottom surgeries" (including, for transmasculine people, removal of organs such as the uterus and ovaries and, in some cases, the construction of a penis and testicles or phalloplasty, and, for transfeminine people, removal of the penis and testicles and the creation of a vagina, clitoris, and/or other parts of the vulva or vulvovaginoplasty), and, for transfeminine people, "facial feminization surgery" and/or tracheal shave procedures. There seems to be some consensus among both medical professionals and trans communities that current vulvovaginoplasty procedures produce "better" outcomes than current phalloplasty procedures. Trans-identified children may take "puberty blockers" to delay the onset of puberty, in order to prevent their bodies from developing "secondary sexual characteristics," which, in turn, may prevent distress and may make medical and surgical transitioning easier later on (Erickson-Schroth 2014; Byne et al. 2012). Although such reports should be taken with a grain of salt, a meta-analysis from 2010 found that about 80 percent of patients who had undergone "hormone therapy" and "sex-reassignment surgery" reported significant improvements in "quality of life." The authors report "demonstrated improvements in gender dysphoria, psychological functioning and comorbidities, lower suicide rates, higher sexual satisfaction and, overall, improvement in the quality of life" (Murad et al. 2010, 214; see also Byne et al. 2012). In general, it appears that only a small percentage of those who undergo "sex-reassignment surgery" express regret (at least publicly) or seek to reverse medical/surgical procedures (Byne et al. 2012), but certainly feminist, queer, and trans communities have an obligation to respect, resource, and support those who seek to "detransition" or "retransition" (Clark 2013; "Detransition | Third Way Trans" n.d.; "REtransition" n.d.).[5]

The history of medical and surgical interventions for trans people in the United States is complex and has been told elsewhere (Meyerowitz 2002). In short, sexologists—Magnus Hirschfield in particular—began to offer trans people hormonal and surgical interventions in the 1910s and 1920s. Christine Jorgensen was the first American to become famous for having undergone "sex reassignment surgery"—traveling to Denmark for treatment and then returning to the United States and speaking publicly about her transition in 1952. In the United States, endocrinologist Henry Benjamin is considered the founder of transition-related health care—supporting hormonal and surgical interventions for trans people—and his 1966 book *The Transsexual Phenomenon* set the standard for transitioning in the United States. In 1979, the Harry Benjamin International Gender Dysphoria Association—now the World Professional Association for Transgender Health (WPATH)—laid out standards of care for treating transgender persons. WPATH continues to update these standards of care regularly, and they are used as guidelines all over the world (Meyerowitz 2002; Stryker 2009; Erickson-Schroth 2014).

In 1980, gender identity disorder (GID) was added as a diagnosis to the American Psychiatric Association's third edition of the *Diagnostic and Statistical Manual of Mental Disorders (DSM-III)*. Some activists and scholars have argued that this diagnosis was added in response to the removal of homosexuality from the *DSM* in 1973, as a way for mental health professionals to continue to pathologize gender and sexual minorities. In particular, some scholars and activists have argued that the inclusion of a "GID" category for children was designed to allow medical providers to attempt to "normalize" gender-atypical children in order to prevent them from growing up to become gay or lesbian adults (Langer and Martin 2004). Currently, the mental health and medical systems are intertwined for trans people seeking transition-related care, as medical and surgical providers often require trans people to receive a mental health diagnosis and to consult with mental health professionals before they will provide hormones or surgery. The GID diagnosis was hotly debated during the most recent *DSM* revision process (from *DSM-IV* to *DSM-5*), with some trans activists seeking complete removal of the diagnosis and some seeking reform but not removal (more on this later). In the *DSM-5*, the diagnosis was changed from "gender identity disorder" to "gender dysphoria" in order to (in theory) emphasize that gender nonconformity is not pathological per se but that some transgender people may experience distress due to the supposed "misfit" between their gender identity and their sexed embodiment (more on distress later). The crafters of the revised category argued that the diagnosis of gender dysphoria would grant legitimacy to and provide justification for insurance coverage of transition-related care for those transgender people who desire medical interventions (Burke 2011; Cohen-Kettenis and Pfäfflin 2009; Zucker 2010). Concern about losing insurance funding for transition-related care was one reason why the working group that devised the diagnosis of gender dysphoria for the *DSM-5* opted not to eliminate a trans-related diagnosis completely (Burke 2011; Sennott 2010; Daley and Mulé 2014).[6]

History of Feminist and Transfeminist Approaches to Transition-Related Care

While strong connections between feminist and transgender movements have existed in the United States since the beginning of the so-called second wave of the U.S. feminist movement (Stryker 2009; Williams 2016), there has also long been a vocal strand of antitrans sentiment among U.S. feminists, and this radical feminist antitrans sentiment has been, in part, related to the medicalization of transgender experience. Most famously, Janice Raymond argued in *The Transsexual Empire: The Making of the She-Male* (1979) that "transsexuals" use the medical system to escape the confines of either masculinity or femininity, rather than dismantling oppressive sex/gender systems entirely (J. G. Raymond 1994), an argument that is still supported by some radical feminists (e.g., Jeffreys 2014). These scholars have tended to argue that medically assisted gender transition itself serves to uphold the gender binary and patriarchal systems of oppression. A somewhat similar argument was made by Bernice L. Hausman in *Changing Sex: Transsexualism, Technology, and the Idea of Gender* (1995), although Hausman is more critical of the medical system and less critical of trans people themselves.

To simplify, in response to the transphobia of Raymond and other feminists, some trans and queer activists and scholars in the 1990s emphasized that trans people experience oppression *because* they are transgender (and not just because of sexist oppression). These scholars and activists also highlighted the ways in which trans people can resist and destabilize gender norms. Like transphobic radical feminists, these scholars and activists did critique the medicalization of transgender experience, focusing on the role of medicine in enforcing gender stereotypes, but did not see transgender experience as synonymous with or limited to the medical model of transsexuality (Stone 1992; Bornstein 1995; Butler 1990, 1993).

In the late 1990s and early 2000s, some trans scholars and activists pushed back against this earlier trans and queer work, arguing (rightly or wrongly) that Judith Butler's work in particular serves to reclaim the "subversive" transgender person who defies gender norms but continues to demonize or exclude the transsexual or transgender person who wishes to use medical interventions to fully "pass" as a man or a woman (see, e.g., Prosser 1998; Namaste 2000; Valentine 2007). Unfortunately, some of this work (especially Jay Prosser's *Second Skins*) defends transsexual experiences by rather essentialist appeals to the body (Prosser 1998; see also Serano 2007).

While I am hesitant to set up a dialectic here or to suggest that trans theorists and activists have successfully resolved the tensions involved in transition-related care, I do believe that contemporary trans scholars and activists have produced generative and nuanced accounts of transition-related medical care—accounts that hold medicine accountable for its normalizing, sexist, racist, imperialist, and neoliberal aspects; that recognize trans people as actors who sometimes uphold, sometimes acquiesce to, and sometimes resist medicine's normalizing imperatives; that affirm the value of medical interventions for those trans people who desire such interventions; and that imagine different—trans-affirming, feminist, queer, crip, antiracist—ways of structuring transition-related care.

Critiques of Medical Approaches to Transition-Related Care

Trans scholars and activists have critiqued the pathologization of trans experience, particularly the inclusion of gender identity disorder (GID) in the *DSM*. These activists and scholars have argued that the diagnosis of GID suggests that gender nonconformity itself is a sign of mental illness, rather than a form of "benign variation" (to use Gayle Rubin's term) (G. Rubin 1984). Thus, according to this critique, the diagnosis of GID has served as a tool for enforcing gender conformity for cis and (especially) transgender people. Some scholars and activists have argued that the diagnosis of GID increases stigma against transgender people; however, it is difficult to make this argument in a way that does not per-petuate stigma against other mental illnesses, a problem that I return to later. As noted above, the change from GID to "gender dysphoria" was intended to address this critique, as the diagnosis of gender dysphoria is not intended to pathologize gender nonconformity per se but only the distress that some trans people experience as a result of the disconnect between their assigned sex/gender and their felt sex/gender; however, critics have argued that the diagnosis for children, in particular, retains its focus on gender nonconformity rather than distress. In addition, to the extent that distress is created by institutionalized transphobia, trans people may still be diagnosed with a mental disorder as a result of social injustice (Burke 2011; Sennott 2010; Daley and Mulé 2014; Tosh 2016).

More pragmatically, a number of activists and scholars have pointed out that trans people are often subject to the drawbacks of pathologization (e.g., stigma) without receiving some of the typical benefits of pathologization. For example, although GID/gender dysphoria is an officially recognized diagnosis, some insur-ance plans in the United States do not cover mental health or medical treatment for GID/gender dysphoria (Sennott 2010; Daley and Mulé 2014; J. M. Dewey and Gesbeck 2017). In addition, the Americans with Disabilities Act (ADA) specifi-cally excludes people diagnosed with GID as a protected category, thus largely preventing transgender people from making federal disability-based rights claims or accessing federal disability-based benefits (an exclusion that some scholars and activists have argued reflects and perpetuates transphobia within the disability rights movement) (Spade 2003; Puar 2015).

Trans scholars and activists have also long argued that medical profession-als have served as gatekeepers to life-saving transition-related care, enforcing antiquated racialized gender norms on transgender people seeking sex/gender-relevant medical interventions. As it currently stands, transgender people seeking medical interventions are often required to prove their "fitness" for "treatment" to mental health providers and doctors before transition-related care is granted. For decades, mental health and medical providers required trans people to describe themselves using the "wrong body" discourse (e.g., I am really a man born in the body of a woman or vice versa). In addition, transmen had to demonstrate a very traditional form of (white, middle-class) masculinity and transwomen had to demonstrate a very traditional form of (white, middle-class) femininity in order to satisfy medical providers. Furthermore, trans people had to be very careful about how they presented their sexuality, and it was often saf-est for trans people to present as relatively "desireless" prior to transitioning and to express the expectation that they would be "fully" heterosexual after transi-tioning. As trans activists and scholars have pointed out, the medical model for transitioning was/is not only sexist and heterosexist but racist and Eurocentric as well, as the vision of masculinity and femininity assumed and promoted by medical providers is a vision of *white* Euroamerican masculinity and *white* Euroamerican femininity—and trans people of all races are expected to conform to this vision. According to trans activists and theorists, while many trans people may embrace these discourses, others who may want to resist these discourses are required to conform to them in order to access medical interventions (J. M. Dewey and Gesbeck 2017; Johnson 2016; Spade 2003; Burke 2011; G. Davis, Dewey, and Murphy 2016; Vipond 2015; Noble 2006).

And it is certainly the case that medicalized understandings of "transsexuality" that were developed in the West have been exported to countries around the world as part of Eurocentric imperialism and colonialism. While Western discourses about transsexuality have not been taken up uncritically in other parts of the world, there is concern that the spread of Western approaches to transsexuality can render "invisible the cultural diversity of gender expressions and identities worldwide" and can impose "an exclusive framework of conceiving gender diversity" (Suess, Espineira, and Walters 2014, 74–75; see also Najmabadi 2008, 2013; Namaste 2011; Stryker 2012).

Due to the hard work of transgender activists and community members, many health care providers who serve trans people are now more flexible about their expectations for trans people. Still, recent studies of medical providers who serve trans people find that these providers continue to serve a gatekeeping and normalizing role. For example, Davis, Dewey, and Murphy (2016) found that providers continue to express sexist and heteronormative beliefs in their approach to intersex and trans patients (G. Davis, Dewey, and Murphy 2016). From a review of medical articles on genital surgeries, Plemons (2014) found that surgeons often still reveal heteronormative beliefs in their goals for surgery (Plemons 2014). Plemons points out that for transwomen, surgeons are most concerned with the vagina, then the clitoris, and then the rest of the vulva, while for transmen, surgeons are most concerned with the penis and then the scrotum. According to Plemons, surgeons are expressly interested in form/appearance—do the genitals "look" normal—and function—generally? Do the created genitals allow for urination, (heterosexual) intercourse, and the experience of (appropriately gendered) sexual pleasure? In addition, the surgeons are implicitly interested in whether the genitals they are creating can "pass muster" in gendered/sexualized social interactions, always imagined in very sexist and heteronormative ways—for example, surgeons want to create "masculine" genitals that can withstand scrutiny in the homosocial space of the locker room (Plemons 2014).[7] Plemons also argues, however, that some transwomen are increasingly focusing on facial feminization surgery (surgeries developed largely with reference to white female faces and notions of white feminine beauty) and deemphasizing genital surgery, based on the idea that in most social situations, the look of one's face is more important in conferring gender than the look of one's genitals. According to Plemons, this change suggests that both transwomen and medical professionals are, to an extent, moving away from a genital-based understanding of sex/ gender (Plemons 2017).

Dewey and Gesbeck (2017) interviewed medical and mental health professionals who specifically identified as trans-affirming and while they found that these providers did try to support the individualized needs and desires of their trans clients without holding them to rigid gender expectations, they still expected trans patients to present as "trans enough," which meant expressing an intense, distressing, and longstanding sense of disidentification with their sex/ gender of assignment. In addition, if trans clients admitted that they were motivated by particular forms of sexual desire (e.g., if they were aroused by "crossdressing"), they could be diagnosed with a paraphilia and denied access to transition-related care.[8] Finally, trans clients were required to demonstrate "mental competence" prior to receiving surgery, thus potentially excluding trans people with cognitive or mental disabilities from receiving care (J. M. Dewey and Gesbeck 2017).

Castañeda argues that current WPATH guidelines for the treatment of "transgender children" also reflect gender-normative commitments; the guidelines recommend, in some cases, administering puberty blockers to trans children. According to Castañeda, medical professionals support the administration of puberty blockers in part because they assume that preventing the onset of puberty will allow trans children to more "perfectly" transition as teenagers or adults, as the puberty blockers will allow doctors to create more gender-normative adults, thus potentially reducing genderqueer forms of being-in-the-world. Castañeda also argues that the guidelines for treating transgender children assume a developmental trajectory—as less mature and more gender-fluid children are expected to develop into more mature and gender-stable adults, thus eliding nondevelopmental perspectives such as those suggested by Jack Halberstam in *The Queer Art of Failure*, in which linear, teleological progress toward "mature adulthood" is rejected in favor of a queer "failure" to develop, reproduce, and/or mature (Castañeda 2015).

In addition to critiquing the way that medical regimes impose sexist, heterosexist, and racist norms on trans people, trans scholars and activists have also critiqued the fact that our society compels trans people to undergo medical interventions, whether desired or not. Transitioning medically/surgically can reduce the stigma, discrimination, and violence faced by trans people. In addition, trans people often must transition medically/surgically in order to access a number of rights and services—including the right to change identification documents (which in turn affects a person's ability to obtain employment and housing and to travel safely) and the right to access appropriate gender/sex-segregated services or facilities—such as public bathrooms, foster group homes, residential drug and alcohol treatment facilities, homeless and domestic violence shelters, and jails and prisons.[9] These requirements differentially affect low-income trans people and trans people of color—who are least able to afford transition-related care but are most likely to need social services and are more likely to be incarcerated. For these reasons, some scholars and activists argue that medical transitioning can in no way be considered a voluntary endeavor (Spade 2011; Silver 2013; Gehi and Arkles 2007).

Drawing on Lisa Duggan's concept of *homonormativity*, trans scholars have used the term *transnormativity* to describe the ways in which certain, highly medicalized, forms of trans experience have achieved some legitimacy in U.S. society (and transnationally), perhaps further marginalizing other forms of trans experience (Duggan 2002). In "Trans Necropolitics: A Transnational Reflection on Violence, Death, and the Trans of Color Afterlife," Snorton and Haritaworn argue, "It is necessary to interrogate how the uneven institutionalization of women's, gay, and trans politics produces a transnormative subject, whose universalized trajectory of coming out/transition, visibility, recognition, protection, and self-actualization largely remains uninterrogated in its complicities and convergences with biomedical, neoliberal, racist, and imperialist projects" (Snorton and Haritaworn 2013, 67).

One strand of this scholarship has focused on the hierarchies that have been created between different forms of trans experience. For example, in a 2015 paper, Austin Johnson argues that "the medical model operates as a normative accountability structure that influences transgender people's experiences of doing gender in multiple institutions of social life including health and healthcare, transgender community groups, and the legal system" (Johnson 2015, 806). In a 2016 paper, Johnson folds this idea of the medical model as a normative accountability structure into the broader concept of transnormativity, which Johnson argues is a set of normative standards—largely based on the medical model—to which all trans people are held accountable. Johnson argues that these normative standards are enforced by multiple institutions, including the medical system, the legal system, and (some) transgender narratives and community groups (Johnson 2016). According to Johnson and others, these normative standards are generally essentialist (based on a "born this way" narrative) and focus on the importance of medical/surgical transition for trans identity (Johnson 2016; Vipond 2015). Vipond, for example, also argues that transnormativity is essentialist, relies on pathologization, creates a hierarchy between "good" and "bad" trans people, and does not account for the racial and economic struggles faced by many trans people (Vipond 2015).

A second strand of this scholarship has focused on the ways that transnormalization entails incorporation into neoliberal and imperialist projects. Susan Stryker and Nikki Sullivan argue that both self-demand amputation (under the label of body integrity identity disorder or BIID) and transsexual genital surgery have been represented and understood as attempts to restore bodily "integrity" and that these procedures can work to integrate previously abjected bodies/selves into the social/political body as productive citizens. For example, they argue that in the 1960s, San Francisco simultaneously began to fund transition-related care and job training for street queens who embraced transsexuality (Stryker and Sullivan 2009). They write, "From the beginning, the mobilisation of a pathologised category of deviant identity—the transsexual—functioned as a means of 'making live' bodies that sovereign power formerly had 'let die'" (Stryker and Sullivan 2009, 60). They go on to suggest that certain forms of sex/gender transition have become a type of "normative transgression" (Stryker and Sullivan 2009; see also Castañeda 2015). Jasbir Puar expands on this discussion in her article "Bodies with New Organs: Becoming Trans, Becoming Disabled" (Puar 2015), arguing that transnormativity reflects ableism—through the idea that trans people can be "cured" through medical/surgical intervention (passing). She goes on to argue, however, that there is a second form of transnormativity that is not about "passing" but is about "piecing"—basically, a form of transnormativity in which the endless plasticity and transformation of the trans body (including through the use of medical technology) fits into or exemplifies broader neoliberal forms of bodily fragmentation for capitalist profit (Puar 2015). Puar also argues that we may be witnessing the development of a type of trans(homo)nationalism, in which racist and imperialist projects co-opt trans rights discourses in order to represent the "tolerant" West as more enlightened than the intolerant, transphobic East (Puar 2015).

Justifying Transition-Related Care

And yet, despite these robust critiques of past and current medical approaches to trans experience, most trans activists and scholars affirm the right of and, in some cases, necessity for trans people to access transition-related medical interventions and have sought to reimagine how these interventions could be better structured to meet the needs of trans people. This task of affirmation and reimagination is a difficult one, as it seeks to answer the question posed by Puar:

> Given that [some] trans bodies are reliant on medical care, costly pharmacological and technological interventions, legal protections, and public accommodations from the very same institutions and apparatuses that functionalize gender normativities and create systemic exclusions, how do people who rely on accessing significant resources within a political economic context that makes the possessive individual the basis for rights claims (including the right to medical care) disrupt the very models on which they depend in order to make the claims that, in the case of trans people, enable them to realize themselves as trans in the first place? (Puar 2015, 47)

Puar answers her own question by advocating for "trans becoming," a concept (like "race racing") that seeks not to eliminate gender differences but rather proliferate and intensify them in order to dissolve binaries through the "over-whelming force of ontological multiplicity" (Puar 2015, 66). Puar herself does not specify what the role of medical interventions would be in this proliferation and intensification, but medical technologies could be used to create a proliferation of differently sexed/gendered forms of mind/bodies, as has been imagined by some trans scholars and activists (see, e.g., Spade 2003) and has been actually practiced by some (see Preciado 2013), even if, in the present and perhaps in the future, sex/gender-relevant medical interventions are primarily used in the service of the sex/gender binary. Puar's model offers a way to think about medical interventions as potential sites of creativity and proliferation, even if she argues that these sites will (almost?) always eventually be coopted by neo-liberal regimes.

While Puar (and others) offer a rationale for medical interventions that dis-solve binaries, other trans scholars have developed rationales for even those med-ical interventions that conform to or reinforce binaries, based on the possibility that medical interventions can alleviate suffering, even suffering that is, in part, socially produced. Trans scholar Alexandre Baril draws on disability studies to develop a model of trans experience that can account for the pain or suffering experienced by some trans people as simultaneously socially produced and, somehow, exceeding the boundaries of the social. Baril identifies within disabil-ity studies the existence of a "composite model of disability" that both critiques social oppressions while recognizing suffering and the possibility that not all suf-fering can be eliminated through societal changes. Baril argues that, for some trans people, trans suffering cannot be reduced to external or internalized cis-genderist oppression and cannot be eliminated entirely through social justice work. Baril writes, "I experience transness in much the same way I experience depression or anxiety; although I know that these states are influenced by struc-tural factors (oppressive systems). . . . Trans suffering can neither be separated from social oppression nor be reduced to it" (Baril 2015, 69).[10]

Baril's article is a useful attempt to combine social constructionist with mate-rialist/phenomenological accounts of trans in a way that acknowledges the dys-phoria experienced by some transgender individuals and the importance of med-ical interventions in some cases. I would suggest, however, that Baril's argument could be further refined based on insights from feminist science studies—Baril suggests that even in a transformed society, there would be some kind of "resid-ual" trans suffering and that this, implicitly, serves as a justification for medical care. However, accepting the insight from feminist science studies that society and mind/body are always already mutually co-constitutive in an iterative fash-ion, I argue that we cannot know in advance whether there would be "residual" trans suffering in an altered society. If society and body/mind are in a co-constitutive relationship, there is not some "residual" aspect of the body/mind that will inevitability resist the effects of societal change.

I argue, instead, that we do not need to agree that there is some kind of trans suffering that exceeds the social in order to justify medical intervention, and in fact, we can remain agnostic about the "biological" causes of gender dysphoria— it may be the case that trans suffering could be eliminated entirely through social transformation at some point in the future (or not), but to the extent that medical interventions are effective in alleviating suffering, they can still be a useful response to mind/body distress. In addition, medical interventions directed at the body/mind could have social, in addition to mind/body, effects, if the mind/body and the social are in constant "intra-action." To put this another way, I argue that if we accept that the social and the biological are mutually constitutive, then any "social" intervention will also be a "mind/body" intervention and any "mind/body" intervention will also be a "social" intervention. There is no a priori reason why socially caused distress must be alleviated by a social intervention; conversely, there is no reason why biologically caused distress must be alleviated by a medical intervention.

IMPROVING TRANSITION-RELATED CARE

From the literature critiquing the current conceptualization and delivery of transition-related care, it is clear that there is much that needs to be reformed about this care in order to make it more trans-affirming, feminist, queer, crip, and antiracist. I offer the following suggestions.

Remove Coercion

Clearly, people should not be coerced into pursuing transition-related care. The conditions that currently make medical/surgical transitioning coercive—from transphobia to making legal rights and social services contingent on medical/surgical transitioning to the very existence of sex/gender-segregated social institutions—must be eliminated. Recognizing that this change may be difficult to achieve and/or a long time in coming, a number of trans activists and scholars have proposed intermediate steps—such as classifying "legal" sex/gender on the basis of "lived" sex/gender, rather than on the basis of assigned sex/gender or evidence of a medical/surgical sex/gender transition (Silver 2013; Spade 2003, 2011).

Validate Multiple Ways of Being/Becoming Trans

As part of eliminating coercion, society must value multiple forms of trans experience, without creating a hierarchy of trans experience that places those who have "fully" medically/surgically transitioned at the top. In one of the introductions to *Trans Bodies, Trans Selves*, Jennifer Finney Boylan lists some of the different ways of being trans, concluding, "There are so many, many ways of being us. If we know anything, it's that trans identity and trans experience are a work in progress, a domain in which the discourse itself is still in a state of evolution and growth" (Erickson-Schroth 2014, xvii). Until recently, only those trans narratives and experiences that fit into the medical model fairly neatly received any significant (if still only partial and tenuous) social support or legitimation, and trans narratives and experiences that departed from the medical model have been ignored or violently erased. Trans activists and allies must work to build a society that fully recognizes, includes, and supports trans people who desire no medical/surgical interventions, who desire to use medical interventions in ways that disrupt standard sex/gender categories (e.g., testosterone plus breast augmentation), who desire certain medical/surgical interventions but not others in order to conform to standard sex/gender categories (e.g., hormone therapy but not genital surgery), and those who desire to use the entire "suite" of available sex/gender-relevant medical interventions in order to conform to standard sex/gender categories. Trans allies must also challenge the idea that Western medical approaches should supersede non-Western sex/gender transition processes in other parts of the world.[11]

Change Gatekeeping Function of Medical Community

Harm Reduction Strategies. In addition, it is absolutely clear that mental health and medical providers must no longer regulate access to transition-related medical care based on gender stereotypes or preconceived notions of who is "trans enough" to deserve care. There is certainly debate within trans communities about how best this can be accomplished. Some activists and scholars have advocated for reform of the psychiatric diagnosis of GID/gender dysphoria, arguing that the diagnosis should focus on distress, not gender nonconformity per se, although it is certainly the case that in a transphobic society, distress may be the result of social stigma and discrimination (Burke 2011).

Other activists and scholars have argued that the diagnosis should be removed from the *DSM* and from the mental/behavioral section of the *International Classification of Diseases* (*ICD*) and should be reconceptualized as a "medical" (as opposed to "psychiatric") condition (Burke 2011; Sennott 2010). This appears to be the position taken by groups like Informed Consent for Access to Trans Health Care (ICATH) and Stop Trans Pathologization (STP). ICATH argues that trans people should not have to receive a psychiatric diagnosis or see a mental health professional before accessing transition-related care. Their website states, "ICATH promotes a departure from the system that uses Gender Identity Disorder Diagnosis and Gender Dysphoria as a means for accessing gender-confirming health care, and follows the Standard of Care already established for non-trans people accessing gender affirming healthcare" ("ICATH" n.d.).[12] ICATH argues that trans people should be able to access transition-related care from doctors according to an "informed consent" model, such that the doctor would provide the trans patient with information about the procedure(s), including risks, and the trans patient would decide for herself/himself/themselves whether to opt for a particular intervention ("ICATH" n.d.).[13] Similarly, STP is an international activist coalition advocating for the removal of gender dysphoria/gender identity disorder from the *DSM* and the *ICD* ("Stop Trans Pathologization—2012" n.d.; Suess, Espineira, and Walters 2014). In 2016, STP published a press release applauding the *ICD*'s proposal to move a trans-specific diagnosis from the chapter on "Mental and behavioural disorders" to a chapter on "Conditions related to sexual health," while continuing to oppose the inclusion of a diagnosis for children and urging the *ICD* to change from what they consider the pathologizing language of "gender incongruence" to a "non-pathologizing and descriptive terminology for the code related to gender transition-related body modification processes in adolescents and adults" (STP—International Campaign Stop Trans Pathologization 2016).

I do not find this proposal to be fully theoretically satisfying, agreeing with Drescher et al. that "while reducing the stigmatization of mental disorders is important, the argument to remove a diagnostic category from the mental disorders section of the ICD simply because mental disorders are stigmatized is neither compelling nor persuasive" (Drescher, Cohen-Kettenis, and Winter 2012). Such a move leaves intact or even heightens the stigmatization of mental illness. In addition, it does not eliminate the gatekeeping function of the medical profession; it simply transfers diagnostic power to medical doctors as opposed to mental health professionals. More broadly, the model of "informed consent" used by ICATH in particular relies on a liberal model of subjectivity and is easily coopted into a neoliberal context in which rational, autonomous "consumers" are expected to "select" the appropriate medical interventions in order to maximize their productivity as citizen/consumers and are held responsible for both medical "successes" and "failures" (for a discussion of informed consent, see Fisher 2013; S. Y. H. Kim 2011; F. Wilson et al. 2014; Brudney 2009).

However, this move does maintain the justification for public funding of transition-related care. In addition, such a move may have important practical benefits for trans people, as it may simplify and increase the affordability of transition-related care (as trans people would not necessarily need to see both a mental health professional and a medical doctor). Thus, this approach could be considered a harm-reduction strategy.[14]

Of course, one option for eliminating the gatekeeping function of the medical profession is to completely eliminate any kind of medical or psychiatric diagnosis for transition-related care. Again, this could potentially reflect and reinforce ableism, if the reason for "demedicalization" is to escape the stigma that comes with any kind of illness, disease, or disorder (not just mental illness). More practically, the major concern with this approach is that, in places like the United States, eliminating any kind of diagnosis for transition-related care could threaten public funding for these medical interventions. Even if some forms of health insurance in the United States do not currently cover transition-related care, it is possible that they might do so in the future (Burke 2011; Giordano 2012). For example, beginning in 2014, Medicare (government health insurance for older Americans) began to cover "medically necessary" hormone therapy and "sex-reassignment" therapy for transgender people, and some Medicaid programs (depending on the state) do as well ("Medicare" n.d.; Gehi and Arkles 2007). The Affordable Care Act (ACA) (2010) in theory prohibited most health insurance providers in the United States from refusing a priori to cover transition-related care ("Healthcare" n.d.). Some activists and scholars are concerned that these existing benefits and the potential to expand these benefits will be lost if transition-related care is completely "demedicalized" (Burke 2011; Giordano 2012). After all, the "gender affirming health care" for cis people cited by ICATH (such as breast augmentation for ciswomen or testosterone injections for cismen)—if not based on a recognized "medical condition" such as hypogonadism—is usually considered "elective" or "cosmetic" and is usually not covered by health insurance. The ciswomen who sought out the services of people like Morris were likely doing so because they could not afford to obtain soft tissue augmentation from a licensed medical provider. This explains, in part, recent (and not always successful) efforts by the medical/ pharmaceutical-industrial complex to develop diagnoses (like "andropause") that could provide a justification for these types of interventions (for a discussion of andropause, see Marshall and Katz 2013).

Another option for democratizing care, not necessarily related to diagnostic reform, would be to expand the orbit of people who could potentially provide certain types of transition-related care. In the United States, interventions like electrolysis are provided by "nonmedical providers," and although it appears to be uncommon, some trans people have been able to get at least some electrolysis procedures covered by health insurance (Jackson n.d.; "Is There Any Way to Get Laser or Electrolysis Covered under Insurance?" n.d.; "Getting Electrolysis Covered" n.d.; "Anyone Have Luck Getting Electrolysis Covered by Insurance?" n.d.). While some surgical procedures must be performed by highly trained medical professionals (including the types of fat tissue transplants and silicone implants that Morris's clients could not afford), I see no reason why "lay health care providers" could not be trained and licensed to prescribe and monitor transition-related hormone therapies. Indeed, as mentioned in the discussion of the Morris case, many trans folks who cannot access mainstream transition-related care rely on illegally obtained hormones, which they self-administer, often following the advice of other trans people. This is not ideal as illegally obtained hormones may not be the correct type or dosage, and there are risks that come with hormone therapy that do need to be monitored. However, this is currently the only option for many trans people (Erickson-Schroth 2014; Weinand and Safer 2015). I see no real reason why nonmedical doctors could not be trained and licensed to provide legal access to hormone therapy. Reducing the level of training required to provide legal hormone therapies could potentially increase the number of providers and reduce costs (which could improve access). In addition, it might allow more trans folks themselves to provide these services legally. While certainly not guaranteed, it seems probable that trans folks are more likely to provide trans-affirming care than nontrans folks. This proposal bears some resemblance to the efforts by some women's health activists to "demedicalize" (but not necessarily deprofessionalize) childbirth by licensing/ obtaining legal recognition for doulas and midwives and to "demedicalize" and "deprofessionalize" abortion by advocating for over-the-counter status for abortion-inducing medication (Coeytaux and Nichols 2014; Lombardo 2015). However, implementing this particular proposal in the United States in regards to hormone therapies may be difficult (even if the strategy pursued is demedicalization but not deprofessionalization), as medical providers are likely to resist "infringements" on their turf and because testosterone, in particular, is regulated as a controlled substance.[15] In addition, it would not improve the accessibility of those interventions that do require significant training and expertise to perform.

I think that eliminating any kind of medical or mental health diagnosis linked to transition-related care without simultaneously (or first) completely transforming how we as a society decide what medical interventions should be covered by insurance (either public or private) may not be worth the risk. Thus, in terms of temporary strategies, I believe that we should focus simultaneously on reforming diagnoses, on educating medical professionals so that they are less likely to hold trans people to heterosexist or "trans enough" standards, and on expanding the orbit of people who are legally allowed to provide transition-related care.

Transformative Possibilities. In terms of a longer-term vision, we must ultimately decide whether we want to base public funding of transition-related care on the argument that transition-related care is medically necessary or on some other justification. As a broader question, I will return to this discussion in the final chapter of the book, but here I will review some of the alternative justificatory discourses that have been proposed for transition-related care.

A number of scholars and activists have argued that transition-related care should be considered a human right. STP members, for example, call for an "elaboration of a human rights–based framework for state-funded coverage of transition-related health care" and point to the Argentinian Gender Identity Law (2012) as establishing a precedent for such an approach (Suess, Espineira, and Walters 2014; for a discussion of the Argentinian law, see Rucovsky 2015). STP, and others, explicitly draw on the feminist framework of reproductive rights as a model, writing, for example, "We take here the words from the feminist movement in their fight for the right to abortion, and the right to your own body: we demand our right to freely decide whether if we want or not to modify our bodies. Our rights to be able to carry on with our decision, with no bureaucratic, political or economical impediments, nor any other type of medical coercion" (International Network for Trans Depathologization n.d.). Similarly, Jamie Lindemann Nelson suggests that transition-related care should be seen as analogous to pregnancy and birth-related care, writing,

> Motherhood is a social role that many people deeply want to occupy. Moreover, many of them want to achieve that role in a way that crucially involves their bodies. Medical assistance in the project is often welcome and sometimes needed to avert poor, or even tragic, outcomes. Yet it is not strictly necessary for becoming a mother. There are analogies here with transgender: while many transgender people see medical interventions as essential for social acceptance and personal integrity, others do not. (J. L. Nelson 2016, 1136)

The connection between reproductive rights and transition-related care certainly makes sense—after all, abortions can be medical procedures, but the feminist demand for abortion rights is not based on the claim that abortions are always medically necessary but on the claim that the right to have an abortion is a necessary component of personal and bodily autonomy (Skinner 2012). In addition, while early feminist arguments for abortion rights focused on the issue of "choice," other feminist frameworks—including reproductive rights and, even more so, reproductive justice frameworks informed by women of color activism and theorizing—have focused on the issue of access—arguing that people must have access to the resources necessary to make and carry out decisions about sexuality, childbearing, and childrearing (Price 2011; D. E. Roberts 2015; Ross and Solinger 2017; A. Smith 2005; Correa and Petchesky 1994). The organization SisterSong, for example, defines reproductive justice as "the human right to maintain personal bodily autonomy, have children, not have children, and parent the children we have in safe and sustainable communities" ("Reproductive Justice" n.d.). Scholars and activists have already begun to conceptualize some trans rights through a reproductive justice framework (see, e.g., Nixon 2013). Conceptualizing transition-related care itself as part of a reproductive justice platform is deeply appealing and connects scholarship and activism related to transition-related care to worldwide, people of color–led movements for justice and freedom.[16] Particularly in a non-U.S. context, the human rights framework has, in some cases, served as an important tool for advancing the agendas of marginalized communities. I certainly support all those who find this approach useful; however, a number of scholars and activists have engaged in complex debates over the value of the human rights framework both in the realm of "women's rights" (e.g., Grewal 1999; Lloyd 2007; Reilly 2007; Nash 2002; D. Collins et al. 2010) and in the realm of "LGBTQ+ rights" (Hines 2009; Waites 2009; Kollman and Waites 2009; Dreyfus 2012). It is beyond the scope of this chapter to fully engage with these discussions. In brief, in addition to concerns that have been raised by feminists about the androcentric, ethnocentric, essentialist, and universalizing character of the human rights framework, queer and trans studies scholars have worried that the human rights framework could consolidate fixed sexual and gender identity categories, thereby precluding sexual or gender fluidity. While arguing for the pragmatic value of a human rights approach to trans rights, Tom Dreyfus suggests that "the 'half-invention' of the category of 'gender identity' [in human rights accords] may unwittingly subject people of diverse gender identities to the discursive production of fixed identities instead of their own conceptions of blurred identification" (Dreyfus 2012, 33).

Given the somewhat fraught nature of arguing for transition-related care based on a "human rights framework," I believe it is worthwhile to develop multiple alternative justificatory discourses. Here I draw on the work of Simona Giordano (2012) to offer one such alternative. Giordano explores possible moral arguments for funding transition-related care if a diagnosis for GID is eliminated. According to Giordano, one could argue that if "GID" is eliminated, transition-related care should be considered "on par" with other body modifications—like cosmetic surgery or "racial" surgery—and should be privately negotiated and paid for. According to Giordano, however, one could also argue that it does not matter whether transition-related care is like other body modifications. Giordano writes,

> The argument that 'because many types of body modifications are matters of private transaction therefore medical treatment for gender dysphoria must also be' is also flawed. It might well be that some other types of body modifications should also be funded publicly or reimbursed under insurance schemes.... This does not mean that all claims to body modifications deserve social support.... Whether or not medical treatment should be offered and paid for depends not on the type of condition one has, but on whether the condition (whether associated with gender, ethnic belonging or others) is severe enough to impinge significantly upon the quality of life of the sufferer, to markedly jeopardize his/her psycho-social functioning, and whether available medical treatment is likely to ameliorate his/her condition. (Giordano 2012, 37)

I would alter Giordano's language somewhat to argue that transition-related care should be publicly supported if/because it is effective, prevents suffering, and enables people to live more fulfilling lives. Of course, in a deeply unjust society, people individually pursuing their own flourishing will almost inevitably lead to the perpetuation, and even strengthening, of racist, sexist, heterosexist, ableist, and transphobia norms and institutions. Thus, as feminist activists, as we allow and perhaps encourage people to pursue their own flourishing, we must also work to transform the broader structures of our society in order to foster justice.

While Giordano does not suggest that their argument might extend beyond transition-related care and body modifications, what I want to argue in the final chapter is that this argument does not just apply to certain types of medical interventions but to all medical interventions—it is unnecessary and even unproductive to argue over whether X is a "real" disease, illness, or disorder in order to decide whether medical interventions should be socially funded. Rather, we should use criteria such as those proposed by Giordano (modified somewhat): primarily, is a particular medical intervention necessarily for a person to live a fulfilling life?

In addition, as will be discussed later, decisions about funding must take into account broader social, political, and economic contexts. We must ask questions such as, even if the intervention promotes an individual's flourishing, will it have negative effects on others or on society? What percent of our social resources should be allocated to medical interventions? The answers to these questions will always be value judgments, influenced by social and cultural norms, and cannot be decided via recourse to "biological" or "objective" facts. And while doctors, researchers, and medical professionals certainly have a role to play in these decision-making processes, their voices are no more important than the voices of a variety of other important constituencies.

Learning from the Case of Transition-Related Care

Contemporary trans scholars and activists have produced generative and nuanced analyses of transition-related medical care—analyses that hold medicine accountable for its normalizing, sexist, racist, imperialist, and neoliberal aspects; that recognize trans people as actors who sometimes uphold, sometimes acquiesce to, and sometimes resist medicine's normalizing imperatives; that affirm the value of medical interventions for those trans people who desire such interventions; and that imagine different, and more just, ways of structuring transition-related care.

The most important insight for this project that comes from the Morris case and from transition-related care more generally is that it is sometimes necessary to hold together contradictory positions. Transition-related care is life-saving, or at least highly beneficial, for many transgender individuals, and we must work to ensure that all trans people who need or want it have access to this care. At the same time, we can recognize that this care, as it is currently configured, is inflected with transnormativity, sexism, heterosexism, racism, class, ableism, and colonialism. More specifically, as it is currently configured, transition-related care is designed to produce gender-normative subjects. If we as a society expand access to transition-related care as it is, we will be reproducing these problematic dynamics. Thus, as trans/feminist activists work to expand access to transition-related care, we must also work to change how this care is configured, and we must work to transform the broader society in which this care is located. The two efforts must be pursued together, even though they are in some ways contradictory and even though, at times, one effort may undermine the other. I argue that this ability to analytically and practically hold together contradiction, found within trans studies and trans activist approaches to transition-related care, is a resource for feminist approaches to medicine more broadly.

CHAPTER 4

Sexuopharmaceuticals

QUEERING MEDICALIZATION

In this chapter, I examine the category of what scholars have called "sexuopharmaceuticals"—drugs used with the intention of altering sexual desire and/or functioning, such as (most famously) Viagra. As noted in the Introduction to this book, it was in attempting to evaluate the ethics and politics of drugs for female sexual dissatisfaction (and the ethics and politics of feminist campaigns to halt the production of these drugs) that I first became "stuck"—unable to decide whether or not I agreed with the efforts of anti-sexuopharmaceutical activists.

A decade later, I still find the arguments offered on both sides to be persuasive. On one hand, critics argue that sexuopharmaceuticals, both as a broader discursive formation and as individual interventions into specific cases of sexual dissatisfaction, largely serve to promote and reinforce phallocentric and heteronormative sexual desires and activities. On the other hand, supporters argue that sexuopharmaceuticals can be used to facilitate queer(er) desires and activities and that, even in cases where they are not used "queerly," they may still promote well-being for some in a society not particularly well designed to promote sexual flourishing. Thus, I argue for directing activist attention away from directly opposing these drugs to working to transform the broader society in order to create the conditions under which multiple forms of sexuality and nonsexuality can flourish.

Before turning to an in-depth analysis of sexuopharmaceuticals, I briefly describe the struggle that occurred over the approval of flibanserin/Addyi (dubbed "the female Viagra" by the media). There were numerous actors—including feminist organizations and activists—involved on both sides of the struggle, and highlighting their participation in this conflict suggests how complicated the issue really was/is. After introducing this conflict, I then offer an examination of sexuopharmaceuticals for "male" sexual dissatisfaction, tracing their history and feminist arguments for and against their use. Then, I return to an examination of sexuopharmaceuticals for "female" sexual dissatisfaction, again tracing their development and examining their ethicopolitical status. I finally turn to some qualitative research that I conducted with asexually identified individuals for an earlier project (Gupta 2013a, 2015a, 2015b, 2017) to shed additional light on this issue. Asexually identified individuals have good reason to oppose sexuopharmaceuticals, especially those intended to increase sexual desire, as the existence of these drugs seems to suggest that a lack of sexual interest or attraction is pathological. However, while most of my interviewees were critical of sexuopharmaceuticals, they still felt that people should be able to access these drugs if their use would promote well-being. I argue that the asexually identified individuals in my study offer the outlines of an ethically and politically responsible answer to the contradictions embedded in the space of sexuopharmaceutical interventions.

Feminists Fighting Over "Female Viagra"

In 2010, a U.S. Food and Drug Administration (FDA) panel recommended against approving flibanserin, a pharmaceutical treatment for "female sexual dysfunction." This decision delighted a group of feminist activists, called the "New View Campaign," who had been organizing against the medicalization of female sexual dissatisfaction since the late 1990s. In addition to questioning the safety and efficacy of flibanserin, the New View Campaign objected to the pathologization of benign female sexual variation and the exclusive focus of medical professionals on the biological causes of female sexual dissatisfaction. Members of the campaign actually testified at multiple FDA hearings against approving these types of drugs (The Working Group on A New View of Women's Sexual Problems n.d.; Tiefer 2006).

The campaign's victory was not permanent, however. A small drug company, called Sprout Pharmaceuticals, took over the process of obtaining approval for flibanserin—renamed Addyi—and they enlisted feminist politicians and organizations to bring pressure to bear on the FDA. According to Reuters, in January 2013, a group of Democratic members of Congress—Debbie Wasserman Schultz, Chellie Pingree, Nita Lowey, and Louise Slaughter—wrote to the FDA to encourage them to use the same standard to evaluate drugs for female sexual disorders as they use to evaluate drugs for male sexual disorders (T. Clarke 2014).

In addition, a number of women's groups, consumer groups, and medical groups—including explicitly feminist organizations like the National Organization for Women (NOW)—met with the FDA to protest their initial rejection of Sprout's application. After their meeting, the groups sent a follow-up letter to the FDA, and some of the groups published a press release urging the FDA to approve flibanserin/Addyi (T. Clarke 2014).[1] The press release lists twelve groups "supporting treatment for women's sexual disorder." The list includes the groups that originally met with the FDA along with four additional groups, including the Black Women's Health Imperative. It is somewhat surprising that the Black Women's Health Imperative signed on to this letter, as the group grew out of the feminist women's health movement, which has historically been critical of institutionalized medicine (Heather and Zeldes 2008).

Unlike the feminist activists of the New View Campaign, these "prodrug" feminist activists argued that it was only fair for women to have access to pharmaceutical treatments for sexual dissatisfaction as men have access to Viagra. These feminists criticized the medical profession for ignoring female sexual pleasure and accused the FDA of paternalistically using more stringent standards to evaluate drugs for women than they used to evaluate drugs for men (T. Clarke 2014).

How is it that feminist women's health activists ended up taking such diametrically opposite positions on this issue? Was one side misinformed or misguided? It is possible that those feminists who supported drug treatments for female sexual dissatisfaction were manipulated into supporting Sprout's bottom line; however, it is my contention that both sides were defending legitimate positions. This conflict was not simply the result of muddled thinking or values but reflected the contradictory reality of medical interventions for both female and male sexual dissatisfaction.

MEDICAL INTERVENTIONS FOR MALE SEXUAL DIFFICULTIES: HISTORY AND SCOPE

"Male" sexual difficulties, and specifically the inability to get or maintain an erection, have long been a source of concern in Western societies (McLaren 2007). In 1980, a number of so-called sexual dysfunctions, including desire disorders, arousal disorders, orgasm disorders, and sexual pain disorders, were incorporated into the third edition of the *Diagnostic and Statistical Manual of Mental Disorders* (*DSM-III*), the diagnostic manual used by the American Psychiatric Association (Irvine 2005).

But during the 1980s and 1990s, some doctors wanted to move away from a focus on the psychological bases of sexual dysfunctions in order to focus on the "physiological" or "organic" bases of sexual dysfunction. These doctors adopted the label "erectile dysfunction" or ED (instead of impotence) to describe male erection problems and emphasized the physiological etiology of ED (Marshall 2006). ED is typically defined as the inability to maintain an erection "sufficient for sexual intercourse" (Mayoclinic.com). In 1998, the FDA approved Pfizer's Viagra (sildenafil citrate) as a treatment for ED. Since the release of Viagra, additional medications for ED have been released, including Levitra (vardenafil) and Cialis (tadalafil) (Bella et al. 2015). Between 1998 and 2005, approximately 27 million men worldwide used Viagra (Padma-Nathan 2006).

Viagra and similar drugs work to enhance muscle relaxation in the penis and blood inflow, thus facilitating the development of an erection (Padma-Nathan 2006).[2] According to Pfizer, Viagra will not lead to an increase in sexual desire and will not cause an erection in the absence of sexual stimulation (Pfizer 2010). ED is typically represented by Pfizer as a problem of nerves or blood vessels in the penis (Pfizer n.d.). If nerves or blood vessels in the penis are "malfunctioning," Viagra's mechanism of action explains why it would be effective in treating ED. Yet, the evidence suggests that Viagra is at least as effective for treating ED of psychogenic etiology as for treating ED of organic or mixed etiology, even when compared to placebo (Goldstein et al. 1998). Given Viagra's mechanism of action, it is not immediately clear, from a medical perspective, why Viagra would treat ED of psychogenic origin effectively. Drawing on insights from feminist science studies, I suspect that Viagra's efficacy in treating ED of psychogenic etiology results from the fact that drugs, placebos, psychology/mind, and penis/body exist in a highly complex network of mutual constitution (see E. A. Wilson 2015).

Researchers within the field of biomedicine have generally been pleased with the efficacy of Viagra. In a review article summarizing research conducted since 2002 into the efficacy and safety of Viagra, Padma-Nathan argues that Viagra has been shown to be effective in increasing "erection hardness and rigidity" in a variety of male populations, including men with various comorbidities. According to supporters, Viagra has also been shown to be safe and well tolerated. Trials have also demonstrated that men who use Viagra report increased "self-esteem, confidence, and sexual relationship satisfaction." Finally, Padma-Nathan argues that Viagra effectiveness can be increased by a variety of measures, primarily "titrating to the maximum dose" (Padma-Nathan 2006).

Similarly, some (heteronormative) studies conducted by researchers within the field of biomedicine have found that the female partners of men treated for ED with Viagra report increased sexual satisfaction. For example, Heiman et al. describe the results of a double-anonymous, placebo-controlled study that investigated the sexual satisfaction of partners of men treated with Viagra. They report that, compared to the partners of men treated with a placebo, the partners of men treated with Viagra "had greater frequency of satisfactory sexual intercourse, an increase in sexual satisfaction assessed by the FSFI [Female Sexual Function Index] and enjoyment assessed by the SFQ [Sexual Function Questionnaire], and improvement in some measures of desirability, arousal, and orgasm" (Heiman et al. 2007, 445).[3]

CRITICAL APPROACHES TO "IMPOTENCE" AND VIAGRA

Researchers from outside of the field of biomedicine who have investigated the experiences of men who have used Viagra and their female partners have reported more mixed results. A team of feminist researchers in New Zealand interviewed thirty-three male Viagra users and twenty-seven female partners of male Viagra users. In an article about men's experiences with Viagra, the team argues that since the development of Viagra, the biomedical community has endorsed the concept of "sex for life," which the authors define as "the imperative to maintain an active youthful masculine [hetero]sexuality—defined in terms of male orgasm through penetrative sex," even in old age (Potts et al. 2006, 306). In a second article, the team focuses on the negative experiences of the female partners of male Viagra users. According to the team, some of the women interpreted the following aspects of Viagra use as unwelcome: increased frequency and duration of sex, sometimes leading to vaginal pain; focus on penile-vaginal intercourse at the expense of other activities; pressure to have sex; disruption of the "normal" aging process; tension and conflict over the use of the drug; fear of a partner's infidelity; and fear of health consequences for their partner. The authors wish to challenge the literature on Viagra in which "Viagra use by men appears to assume an unproblematic link between successful penile erection (and penetration) and user, partner and sexual relationship satisfaction" (Potts et al. 2003, 699).

Feminist scholars have offered a number of important critiques of biomedical understandings of erectile dysfunction and of Viagra (Marshall 2006; Baglia 2005; Potts et al. 2004; Tiefer 2004; Loe 2001; Preciado 2013).[4] I find the following critiques highly persuasive: first, Viagra may not be the most effective solution for many cases of sexual dissatisfaction. The marketing of Viagra suggests that erectile dysfunction is entirely a biological problem and is thus best addressed through a biomedical intervention. However, in some (or many) cases, sexual skills training, relationship counseling, and/or consciousness raising may actually improve sexual satisfaction more than Viagra. However, with the marketing of Viagra, the media attention around Viagra, and the willingness of many health insurance companies to pay for Viagra, these alternatives may not even be considered or, worse, may be considered illegitimate.

Second, as a result of the marketing and availability of Viagra, people with penises (PWPs) (and/or their partners) may feel unwanted pressure to maintain regular sexual activity, specifically penetrative sexual activity, throughout the life course. PWPs (and/or their partners) who would prefer to allow sexual activity to cease or who would prefer to explore alternative sexual practices may feel stigmatized or dysfunctional. In addition, because our society privileges penile-vaginal sexuality, some PWPs (and/or their partners) would never consider exploring alternative types of sexuality unless pushed to do so as a result of erectile dysfunction. Some PWPs (and/or their partners) who explore alternative types of sexuality as a result of impotence may ultimately find these types of sexuality more pleasurable than penile-focused sexuality and may even go on to challenge the societal privileging of penile-focused sexuality (for an example of this, see Kerner 2004).[5] Viagra may foreclose these possibilities for experimentation. Jay Baglia expresses one version of this critique when he writes, "As a reinscription of heterotopia's penile-vaginal penetration, the arrival of Viagra may in fact be stalling the potential for new models of male sexuality" (Baglia 2005, 4). He continues, "As the couple's solution to the couple's disease, Viagra obstructs the possibilities for sexual improvisation . . . I must question the ways in which biomedicine might stall sexual experimentation and elaboration insofar as it ruthlessly excludes the possibilities of sexual variation" (Baglia 2005, 93).[6]

Third, the marketing of Viagra may serve to reinforce the connection between masculinity and the erect penis. A number of Viagra advertisements position ED as a loss of masculinity and Viagra as a way to restore masculinity. Viagra/ED discourse thus equates successful masculinity with the penis and virility as such, a longstanding and very old definition of patriarchal power that has been critiqued by feminists as well as scholars in masculinity, trans, and queer studies. Most PWPs will experience at least a few instances of unwanted penile flaccidness over the course of their lives; if this is understood as preventing "real" sexual activity and undermining masculinity, it may cause some male-identified people (and their partners) unnecessary anxiety. At the same time, reinforcing the connection between masculinity and the erect penis further ties masculinity to a particular form of embodiment, thereby undermining other forms of masculinity, such as some transmasculinities (Baglia 2005; Loe 2001).

Fourth, Viagra can prop up (literally and figuratively) phallocentrism—a type of sexuality that, in general, may be more satisfying for heterosexual men than for heterosexual women. According to this critique, men and women may be mismatched in their levels of interest in penetrative intercourse, especially later in life. Although a couple's sexual life may be the product of negotiation between the two partners, as feminists have pointed out, men may enjoy unearned advantages in the negotiation process. For example, beginning early in their lives, many women have been discouraged from expressing their own sexual desires and have been taught to believe that it is their responsibility to satisfy their partner's sexual wants (often represented as "needs"). Nicola Gavey's work has demonstrated that in many heterosexual relationships, the man's sexual desires often play a larger role in determining the couple's sexual life than the woman's (Gavey 2005). According to this argument, the availability of Viagra can allow men to use their unearned negotiating advantage to make penetrative intercourse a central part of a couple's sexual relationship throughout the life course, contrary to the desires of some women.

Finally, although many feminist analyses of Viagra have not paid adequate attention to the issue of race, an intersectional analysis suggests that the conceptualization and marketing of Viagra reflects and perpetuates a racist, in addition to heterosexist, sexual imaginary. In the United States, black men in particular are often viewed as hypersexual and sexual predators, threatening the purity of white womanhood through rape (Freedman 2013) and the health of black womanhood through the transmission of sexually transmitted infections (STIs), particularly HIV/AIDS (McCune 2014). In thinking about the Viagra "user," medical professionals and the public at large are undoubtedly conceptualizing a white man. It is unlikely that there would be such widespread support or enthusiasm for enabling the phallic sexuality of black men. Indeed, some scholars have noted that few advertisements for Viagra in the United States feature men of color (Botz-Bornstein 2011), and in an analysis of sexual health discourses, Linwood J. Lewis found that research on minority sexual health primarily focuses on preventative sexual health with little attention to the attainment of sexual pleasure (Lewis 2004).[7]

In the category of critiques that I find unpersuasive is the argument that Viagra disrupts the so-called natural process of aging and so-called natural male sexuality. Robert MacDougall's article, "Remaking the Real Man: Erectile Dysfunction Palliatives and the Social Re-Construction of the Male Heterosexual Life Cycle," offers an example of this argument. In this article, when discussing the rise of pharmacological treatments for depression, MacDougall writes, "With prescription in hand, and his synaptic vesicles now teeming with paroxetine and other serotonin reuptake inhibitors, the young man will undoubtedly feel better, but that feeling of contentment will in a very real sense be *simulated*— that is to say, not genuine, because it is not grounded in his phenomenal lifeworld" (MacDougall 2006, 83, emphasis added). Of sexuopharmaceuticals, he writes, "A phenomenon driven by science, commerce, self-importance, and pride may fundamentally change the nature of human intimacy such that we may get to the point when it will be difficult to say what is *real* and what is not" (MacDougall 2006, 85, emphasis added). In these instances, MacDougall reinforces a distinction between phenomenological experience as real, natural, and genuine and chemical processes in the body (including neurochemical processes) as unreal and simulated. This understanding of medicalization is clearly flawed, even by the logic of social constructionism. There was not at some point a pure or natural aging process or a male sexuality not influenced by technology or societal norms that has now become artificial or simulated through technologization. As suggested by feminist science studies, male sexuality has always been the product of an "intra-action" between biology and society, and for centuries, men have used different technological interventions in order to alter penile functioning (McLaren 2007).

IN DEFENSE OF VIAGRA?

Queer theory encourages us to recognize that, in addition to facilitating heteronormative pleasures, Viagra has been used to facilitate all sorts of queer pleasures, including solo and partnered masturbation, oral sex, heterosexual anal sex, sex work of various kinds, and penetrative sex between men, just to name a few. The use of Viagra (and other drugs for erectile dysfunction) for sex work and for penetrative sex between men is not unproblematic. Many scholars and researchers have argued that gay men may use Viagra primarily to counteract the effects of other "recreational" drugs, which, in turn, may be used to counteract the pain caused by a heterosexist society. Recreational drug use can increase a person's risk of contracting HIV/AIDS and other sexually transmitted infections (Díaz, Heckert, and Sánchez 2005; Halkitis and Green 2007; Swearingen and Klausner 2005). However, in *Pleasure Consuming Medicine: The Queer Politics of Drugs* (2009), Kane Race argues that some (or many) gay men who take recreational drugs as part of a gay or queer community use these drugs to produce (potentially queer) pleasure in ways that incorporate both self- and other-directed practices of care and attention. Race writes, "We can nonetheless see that drugs are linked to specific practices of pleasure and forms of sociability. They are used to produce particular contexts of interaction, pleasure, and activity. . . . Most importantly, we can see that specific practices of care and attention are being brought to the question of how to use drugs, such that considerations of safety appear as part of a concern to maximize pleasure, rather than standing in direct opposition to it" (Race 2009, 153–154). This is, of course, an enormously complex issue, and I will simply reiterate that viewing Viagra through a queer lens can allow us to see the ways in which individuals and communities appropriate biomedical technologies in order to facilitate a variety of queer pleasures.[8]

It is certainly true that the broader discursive formation of Viagra (including advertisements, Viagra education focused at doctors, etc.), as well as many individual uses of Viagra, will generally promote phallocentric heteronormativity. Still, even in these cases, we cannot assume that men are simply using Viagra to meet their sexual desires at the expense of their female partners. According to the team of researchers mentioned above, twelve of the men they interviewed challenged the "sex for life" paradigm. Instead, these men talked about their "shifting sexual priorities, goals, and practices; the increasing importance of mutual enjoyment and involvement of partners; and experimentation with alternative sexual practices and pleasures" (Potts et al. 2006, 316).

In addition, these researchers found that all of the women they interviewed were able to negotiate the incorporation of Viagra into their lives at least to an extent (Potts et al. 2003). They write, "Some women were able to resist such pressures [to have penile-vaginal sex on demand] and to negotiate openly with men about when they felt like having sex, what kinds of sex they enjoyed, and when Viagra would be used" (Potts et al. 2003, 714). Also relevant is Sherry Hite's study of female sexuality, as she discovered that while most heterosexual women find it easier to achieve orgasm through external pubic or clitoral stimulation, some women are able to achieve orgasm through penile-vaginal intercourse alone, and many of the heterosexual women in her study reported enjoying penile-vaginal penetration as one part of a sexual encounter that also includes external pubic or clitoral stimulation (Hite 2011). Although we might ask how these (hetero-normative) desires and pleasures have been shaped by social forces, this does not necessarily render these desires (or the dissatisfaction caused by their frustra-tion) illegitimate or unworthy of support. There may be cases where Viagra or similar drugs allow people of all genders to gain more satisfaction from their sexual lives.

A Queer Feminist Approach to Viagra

I argue, therefore, that a queer feminist approach to Viagra should focus on addressing the larger structural problems identified in many of the critiques mentioned above, while at the same time acknowledging the ways in which Viagra can be used to facilitate a variety of sexual pleasures. The critiques of Viagra suggest that we must change the social and cultural context in which Viagra is used by: challenging the idea that sexual activity is necessary for health or happiness while arguing for the pleasures of nonsexuality; challenging the societal privileging of penile-vaginal penetrative intercourse while arguing for the pleasures of other types of sexual activities; challenging the idea that sexual dissatisfaction is always and only an organic problem best addressed through biomedical interventions while arguing for the value of psychological, relational, and political approaches to addressing sexual dissatisfaction; challenging the connection between masculinity and the erect penis while working to expand the boundaries of socially acceptable performances of masculinity; challenging racist stereotypes about the sexuality of people of color that undermine their pur-suit of sexual autonomy and pleasure; and challenging the assumption that het-erosexual women are responsible for meeting the sexual needs of their male part-ners while also empowering women to identify, articulate, and negotiate for their own sexual wants.

Biomedical Approaches to Female Sexual Dissatisfaction: History and Scope

Given the perceived success of pharmaceutical treatments for ED, doctors and pharmaceutical companies became interested in developing drugs to treat women's sexual problems. As in the case of male sexual dissatisfaction, some in the medical and psychiatric communities were not satisfied with existing nosol-ogies for female sexual dissatisfaction in the *DSM* because they felt that the categories overemphasized the psychological bases of sexual dysfunction, as opposed to the organic bases of sexual dysfunction. Beginning in 1997, research-ers, clinicians, and drug company representatives met in a series of closed

conferences, financed by the pharmaceutical companies, to discuss the issue. The
1998 conference produced a consensus report defining female sexual dysfunction (FSD) as a collection of sexual dysfunctions (Irvine 2005; J. R. Fishman 2004;
Hartley 2006; J. Drew 2003). The consensus report retained the four major categories of dysfunction from the *DSM-IV* (desire, arousal, orgasm, and pain disorders) but expanded the definitions to include physical as well as psychological
causes of female sexual dysfunction (Basson et al. 2000).[9]

Viagra was tested in women with female sexual arousal disorder (the subset
category of FSD believed to be the rough female equivalent of ED), but it was
not effective. In one study, Viagra was shown to increase physiological arousal
(as measured by instruments) but not subjective arousal (as reported by the
women themselves) (Laan et al. 2002). After a large study involving 781 women,
researchers concluded that only certain populations of women would be likely
to benefit from Viagra (Basson et al. 2002).[10] In 2004, Pfizer stopped large-scale
testing of Viagra in women, although they continued to fund small-scale studies
(Mayor 2004; Nurnberg et al. 2008).[11]

After it became apparent that targeting the subcategory of female arousal
disorders would not be a very effective strategy for addressing female sexual dissatisfaction, researchers and drug companies shifted their attention to the subcategory of female desire disorders (hypoactive sexual desire disorder [HSDD]).
Thus, in this case, the focus on desire disorders was less motivated by a particular theory about sexual dissatisfaction than it was motivated by the search for
conditions that could be treated by pharmaceutical interventions. This later
research initially focused on the possibilities of androgen-replacement therapy
(testosterone) for female desire disorders (Hartley 2006, 367). In 2004, Proctor
and Gamble (P&G) applied to the FDA for approval for Intrinsa, a testosterone
patch designed to treat female desire disorders in surgically postmenopausal
women (women who have had their ovaries surgically removed). The FDA Advisory Board recommended not granting approval to Intrinsa, citing long-term
safety concerns and arguing that Intrinsa produced only small benefits. As a
result, P&G withdrew its application to the FDA (Kingsberg 2005; Guay 2005;
DTB 2009). Intrinsa is currently approved for use in some parts of Europe. In
2009, the *Drug and Therapeutic Bulletin* of the *British Medical Journal* reviewed
the current research on Intrinsa. The authors acknowledged that Intrinsa has
demonstrated efficacy in clinical trials, as women taking Intrinsa reported an
additional one to two sexual events (not limited to penile-vaginal intercourse)
per month and increased levels of sexual desire and satisfaction.[12] However, the
authors did not recommend Intrinsa for female sexual desire disorders because
of long-term safety concerns, small improvements in sexual measures and large
placebo responses, and a high incidence of side effects such as acne and hirsutism (unwanted hair growth). In addition, the authors argued that "the evidence

linking low testosterone concentrations to sexual dysfunction in women is inconclusive" (DTB 2009, 30).[13]

As mentioned at the beginning of this chapter, in 2010, the German pharmaceutical company Boehringer Ingelheim applied to the FDA for approval of flibanserin as a treatment for desire disorders in premenopausal women. Flibanserin is a drug that affects neurotransmitters, including serotonin. It was originally tested as an antidepressant but was not effective. In clinical trials conducted by Boehringer Ingelheim, women taking flibanserin reported an additional 0.7 "sexually satisfying events" per month but did not report increases in sexual desire. Women also reported significant side effects from taking the medication. In 2010, the FDA advisory committee recommended against FDA approval for flibanserin, citing a lack of overall efficacy and worrying side effects. Boehringer Ingelheim decided to cease development of flibanserin (Moynihan 2010a, 2010b; Lenzer 2010). A small company, Sprout Pharmaceuticals, subsequently acquired flibanserin. In 2013, Sprout reapplied to the FDA for approval for flibanserin, submitting data from fourteen new clinical studies with an additional 3,000 new patients. The FDA responded with a letter, again declining to approve flibanserin. Sprout appealed this decision, and at the beginning of 2014, the FDA responded, asking Sprout to complete three small additional trials (T. Clarke 2014). In 2015, Sprout resubmitted to the FDA, and the FDA eventually approved flibanserin—now called Addyi—with several restrictions, including a boxed warning about potential side effects and a requirement that Sprout conduct additional tests on the interaction between alcohol and Addyi. In 2016, Sprout and Addyi were purchased by Valeant Pharmaceuticals, and Valeant agreed to refrain from consumer advertising for eighteen months. Thus far, sales of Addyi have been minimal, and the National Women's Health Network (NWHN) has criticized Valeant for not completing FDA-required studies (FDA 2015; Joffe et al. 2016; National Women's Health Network [NWHN] 2016).

FEMINIST APPROACHES TO FEMALE SEXUAL DYSFUNCTION: STRENGTHS AND LIMITATIONS

As suggested at the beginning of this chapter, a number of feminist activists and scholars, including those working with the New View Campaign, have been very critical of the definition of female sexual dysfunction and of pharmaceutical company efforts to develop "treatments" for FSD (Tiefer 2003, 2006; Irvine 2005; Jutel 2010). Not surprisingly, many of the feminist critiques of FSD echo earlier feminist critiques of ED and Viagra. Expanding on the work of these feminist critics, here I outline the problems with defining sexual disinterest as a mental disorder based on feminist concerns: first, FSD as a discursive formation may lead some women to reinterpret a benign variation in their level of sexual interest as a pathological condition in need of treatment. Second, FSD as a discursive formation suggests that there is some objectively healthy level of sexual desire, but the labeling of some level of desire as "too little" or "too much" reflects both social norms and the personal values of clinicians. Third, FSD as a discursive formation allows medical professionals to expand their control over women's sexuality. Fourth, FSD as a discursive formation gives license to drug companies to develop pharmaceutical treatments for sexual disinterest. As drug companies are motivated by profit, they may encourage consumers to take ineffective or risky drug treatments. Drug treatments that have been approved by the FDA to treat specific conditions in specific populations may be marketed and prescribed to people outside of these populations "off label." Fifth, FSD as a discursive formation may privilege men's sexuality. Heterosexual women may feel pressure to meet the sexual desires of a male partner and may feel distress if they do not live up to societal or partner expectations, which would render them vulnerable to receiving a diagnosis of FSD. Sixth, a lack of interest in sex may be the result of a wide variety of factors, including relationship conflict, lack of sexual health education, tiredness due to overwork, and so on. It is suspect to diagnose women who experience a lack of interest in sex as a result of these factors with a mental or medical disorder. And, finally, FSD as a discursive formation may lead to a focus on the individual. Doctors and other medical professionals identify the problem "in" the person and attempt to solve the problem by "fixing" the person, through therapy or medication. This focus on the individual may foreclose attempts to address the relational and societal factors (including sexism) that play a role in producing sexual dissatisfaction.

As in the case of Viagra, feminist scholars and activists have not adequately analyzed the category of race or class in the case of pharmaceutical treatments for female sexual dissatisfaction, but an intersectional analysis suggests that similar racial and class dynamics are at play in both cases. As historians have noted, social and medical concern with "too little" female sexual desire, arousal, and/or satisfaction has generally only arisen in regards to white, heterosexual middle-class women, while social and medical concern about the sexuality of poor women, women of color, and lesbians has generally focused on their "excessive" hypersexuality (Cryle and Moore 2012; Groneman 2001). We can imagine that those who are concerned about female arousal disorders and female desire disorders are again (perhaps unconsciously) imagining their potential beneficiaries as white, middle-class women. This kind of dynamic is apparent in Sarah Ruhl's contemporary play In the Next Room (or the vibrator play), which is based on Rachel Maines's book The Technology of Orgasm (2001). In the play, set in the late nineteenth century, the upper-class white female characters are treated for hysteria through the use of vibrators. The white women in the play are initially unaware that they are experiencing sexual orgasms as a result of using the vibrators, although the main female character undergoes a sexual awakening during the course of the play. In contrast, the one working-class/of color female character in the play—who works as a wet-nurse for one of the white women—is the only female character who seems to know what orgasms are and who apparently experiences orgasms during sex with her husband (Ruhl 2010). This belief that middle-class white women are the ones who suffer from sexual dissatisfaction, while working-class women and women of color are sexually satisfied and knowledgeable about sexuality, likely forms part of the backdrop against which contemporary discourses about female sexuopharmaceuticals are played out, although a few studies have focused on racial and ethnic differences in female sexual dissatisfaction (e.g., Huang et al. 2009), and some of the advertising developed for flibanserin did feature (light-skinned) women of color.[14]

In addition to challenging purely medical approaches to female sexual dissatisfaction, the New View Campaign has also developed an alternative classification system for women's sexual problems. The campaign defines women's sexual dissatisfaction as "discontent or dissatisfaction with any emotional, physical, or relational aspect of sexual experience." According to the campaign, women's sexual dissatisfaction can be categorized based on whether it arises from sociocultural, political, or economic factors; from relationship problems or problems relating to a partner; from psychological factors; or from medical factors (The Working Group on a New View of Women's Sexual Problems n.d.). Importantly, this approach acknowledges the potential role of social, relational, psychological, and biological factors in the production of sexual dissatisfaction and opens the door to multimodal approaches for addressing sexual dissatisfaction, from political activism, to sexual health education, to therapy, to, potentially, drug interventions. However, as suggested earlier, the New View Campaign has generally adopted a skeptical attitude toward medical interventions to address sexual dissatisfaction, focusing its efforts on critiquing Big Pharma rather than on envisioning ways to incorporate medical approaches into a feminist response to sexual dissatisfaction.

Some of these feminist critiques of FSD have suffered from a few important limitations. For one thing, some feminist scholars and activists have failed to recognize the differences between Viagra (and other treatments for erectile dysfunction) and the pharmaceutical treatments developed for FSD. For example, Jennifer Drew argues that the definition of FSD is characterized by phallocentrism, which she defines as the belief that sexuality is limited to "a normal sexual script starting with arousal and foreplay and culminating in the act of sexual intercourse with the man ejaculating into a passive vagina" (J. Drew 2003, 91). It is certainly true that the makers of Viagra probably intended it to facilitate heterosexual penetrative intercourse (although, as I have argued above, it may actually be used to enable a number of different sexual activities involving the erect penis) and that the marketing of Viagra has largely focused on its role in enabling heterosexual penetrative intercourse. However, it is less clear that the developers of different pharmaceutical treatments for FSD have been so focused on penetrative intercourse. For example, in the clinical trials for Intrinsa, researchers measured the number of sexual events women engaged in, but the meaning of "sexual event" was not confined to penile-vaginal intercourse (Kingsberg 2005). In addition, Rosemary Basson was very involved in the definition of FSD. Basson has become known for arguing that some women may not follow a linear sexual script proceeding from desire to arousal to intercourse but may choose to participate in sexual activities for reasons not related to desire or arousal and then develop desire and/or arousal during the course of a sexual encounter (Basson 2000; for a critique of Basson's model, see Tyler 2008). Thus, it may be inaccurate to label FSD as phallocentric. Nonetheless, not surprisingly, the development of drug treatments for FSD has certainly reflected heterosexism—to my knowledge, the women who participated in drug trials for Intrinsa and flibanserin were all engaged in long-term heterosexual sexual relationships. In addition, while neither Intrinsa nor flibanserin/Addyi has yet been marketed in the United States, some advertising that was developed for flibanserin is heterosexist (featuring only heterosexual couples) and is directed primarily at women in long-term relationships.[15]

Yet, this leads me to a second limitation of some feminist approaches to FSD—these approaches have not appreciated the fact that, just as Viagra has been used in more ways than it was probably intended to be used, women might use drug treatments developed for FSD to facilitate a variety of different types of sexuality and sexual activities. Many women may use drug treatments for FSD to facilitate penetrative heterosexual intercourse within the context of a long-term relationship, which, as I have argued about Viagra, is not illegitimate or valueless, but some women may use drug treatments for FSD to facilitate nonpenetrative sexual activities, to facilitate sexual activity outside the context of a long-term relationship, and/or to facilitate same-sex sexual activities. Again, as I have argued in the case of Viagra, I contend here that insights from queer studies should lead us to appreciate the ways in which individuals and communities might appropriate technologies in order to facilitate a variety of sexual—and possibly queer—pleasures.

In addition, whether intended or not, the effect of initial feminist activism around FSD has been to single out female sexuality as an area in special need of protection, an issue raised by those feminist organizations like the National Organization for Women and the Black Women's Health Imperative that urged the FDA to approve flibanserin/Addyi. There are many efficacy and safety issues with Viagra, but it remains an option for men (although, arguably, Viagra is much more effective for treating ED than Addyi is for treating FSD). In addition, the FDA has approved the use of testosterone as a treatment for men for what has been called "androgen deficiency syndrome," again, despite major questions about its safety and efficacy and about whether androgen deficiency syndrome is an actual problem requiring intervention (Coates 2005). While it is not clear whether drugs for female sexual dissatisfaction should be subjected to less review or drugs for male sexual dissatisfaction should be subjected to more review, arguably activism by the New View Campaign has contributed to a situation where female sexuality is receiving differential treatment and heightened protection from the FDA and the media.

Yet, although the feminist activists who wanted the FDA to approve flibanserin/Addyi made a number of valid points, to me their platform is much more limited than the platform of the New View Campaign. Nowhere in the group letter or the press release developed by these "pro-Addyi" activists is there a critique of medical approaches to sexual dissatisfaction or a discussion of larger structural issues; rather, the groups involved simply argue that because drug treatments have been approved for men, they should be approved for women as well. They thus endorse pharmaceutical interventions for female sexual dissatisfaction without challenging either the systemic problems that lead to female sexual dissatisfaction or the sexism, racism, classism, heterosexism, and ableism of the medical system. Thus, while I believe feminist activists on both sides of the debate defended important positions, ultimately I find neither of their platforms to be completely satisfying.

Asexy Approaches to FSD and Hypoactive Sexual Desire Disorder (HSDD)[16]

In recent years, a number of individuals have begun to explicitly identify as asexual and to form online asexual communities. The largest online community, the Asexual Visibility and Education Network (AVEN), was founded in 2001. Although definitions vary, people who identify as asexual often define asexuality as a lack of sexual attraction to other people. According to AVEN's website, "There is considerable diversity among the asexual community; each asexual person experiences things like relationships, attraction, and arousal somewhat differently" (Asexual Visibility and Education Network n.d.). A significant percentage of individuals who identify as asexual also identify as "romantic," indicating that they seek romantic but nonsexual intimate relationships. A number of those who identify as romantic also identify as gay, lesbian, bisexual, and/or panromantic. Some individuals who identify as asexual engage in sexual activity. Motivations for engaging in sexual activity can include curiosity or desire to please a partner, among others.

Because pharmaceutical company efforts to address FSD eventually focused on female desire disorders, these efforts also potentially have repercussions for asexually identified people, as "desire disorders" as a discursive formation seems to suggest that a lack of interest in sexual activity is somehow pathological. Some scholars, including C. J. DeLuzio Chasin (Chasin 2011) and Lori Brotto and

Morag Yule (Brotto and Yule 2009, 2011), have explored the implications for asexually identified people of the definition of hypoactive sexual desire disorder (HSDD) in the revised fourth edition of the *Diagnostic and Statistical Manual of Mental Disorders (DSM-IV-TR)* (American Psychiatric Association 2000).[17] In general, the inclusion of a desire disorder in the *DSM* may encourage others, including doctors and mental health professionals, to view asexuality as a mental disorder. In theory, the fact that a person's lack of sexual desire was supposed to cause "marked distress or interpersonal difficulty" before being diagnosed with HSDD should have prevented individuals who identify as asexual from being diagnosed with a desire disorder. However, a person may only feel distress about a lack of sexual desire because of social stigma, in which case it would be suspect to diagnose that person with a mental disorder. In addition, the inclusion of a "desire disorder" in the *DSM* may itself promote the idea that individuals who identify as asexual are mentally disordered, and if this produces distress, the inclusion of a desire disorder in the *DSM* may actually create the "disorder" it merely seeks to name. Finally, according to the *DSM-IV-TR*, a person could have been diagnosed with a desire disorder if a lack of sexual desire produced "interpersonal difficulties," but it would have been suspect to diagnose one person with a mental disorder merely due to differences between two (or more) partners in their levels of interest in sex.

A petition created by the New View Campaign asking the FDA to deny approval of a drug treatment for female sexual dissatisfaction was circulated on the AVEN website, enlisting asexual activists in the cause. While the *DSM* was being revised (from the *DSM-IV-TR* to the *DSM-5*), asexual activists also developed a report on the definition of HSDD found in the *DSM-IV-TR* and submitted it to the chair of the *DSM-5* working group on sexual dysfunctions. In the report, the authors point out the negative implications of the *DSM-IV-TR*'s definition of HSDD for individuals who identify as asexual.[18] In the report, the authors do not recommend eliminating HSDD entirely. They suggest that there may be individuals for whom low sexual desire is distressing and who might benefit from medical and psychiatric treatment. According to the authors, a well-designed diagnosis could help facilitate treatment for these individuals. The primary suggestions of the report are to (1) include "attraction to neither males nor females"[19] as a sexual orientation category in the *DSM*, (2) require that the lack of sexual desire causes distress to the person and not only "interpersonal difficulties" in order for a diagnosis to be made, and (3) add a clause specifying that the diagnosis of HSDD only applies to people who do not consider themselves asexual. These proposals aimed to reduce the pathologization of people who identify as asexual but are limited by some ableist conceptual moves. Rather than challenging stigma against mental illness and asexuality together, the report seeks to separate asexuality from HSDD in order to avoid associating asexuality with the stigma of mental illness. The stigma against mental illness is left intact and unquestioned. However, in many ways, the report is generous in its efforts to envision a world in which asexuality is accepted as a potentially ful- filling way of being in the world *and* in which people who do not consider them- selves asexual and who are distressed by their lack of sexual desire may receive recognition and treatment.[20]

As part of my research into contemporary asexual identities, I interviewed thirty self-identified asexual individuals, recruited from AVEN.[21] Although a diverse group in some ways, most of my interviewees shared a broadly similar commitment to reducing the stigma associated with asexuality while support- ing the potential value of medical labels and treatments in some cases. Many of my interviewees had found their lack of interest in sex to be distressing at one point or another, both because of stigma and because of the difficulties it had created in relationships. As a result, around one-third of my interviewees had, at one point, consulted a medical or mental health professional in an effort to find an explanation for their asexuality or in an effort to increase their level of interest in sex. Most of these interviewees eventually decided not to pursue these efforts, instead choosing to accept their level of interest in sex. Around half of my interviewees reported some experience of pathologization—in other words, a medical professional, family member, or friend had labeled them disordered even though they themselves were satisfied with their level of sexual interest.

Many of my interviewees specifically rejected the description of asexuality as a pathological condition, instead describing their own asexuality as simply a different way of being-in-the-world. In addition, a number of my interviewees talked about how their particular way of being-in-the-world had enabled them to develop certain valuable capacities. For example, some interviewees felt their asexuality had enabled them to explore nontraditional types of relationships, while others felt their asexuality had led them to become more open-minded and accepting of difference. Thus, my interviewees at least implicitly critiqued the idea that sexual disinterest should automatically be considered a mental or phys- ical disorder, especially in the absence of distress. Some explicitly critiqued the definition of HSDD in the *DSM-IV*, noting, for example, that people could be diagnosed with HSDD if they experienced "interpersonal difficulties" as a result of their disinterest in sex (a criterion that many of my interviewees would have met). In addition, some interviewees leveled critiques against the pharmaceuti- cal industry for their rush to find pharmaceutical treatments for all sorts of human problems. For example, one interviewee said, "Drug companies do have a tendency to try to medicalize all kinds of things. . . . And then they sell you some chemicals with a bunch of side effects to fix whatever that is. And they make money and you get to risk your health."

However, despite their experiences of unwanted pathologization, and despite the fact that most rejected the language of pathology when describing their own disinterest in sex, almost all of my interviewees supported the availability of medical approaches to sexual disinterest. According to my interviewees, individuals who are distressed by their level of interest in sex should be able to take on a diagnostic label like HSDD and seek treatment for HSDD if they so desire. One interviewee's comments on this issue are fairly representative: "I'm totally happy with myself the way I am now, but I could see if someone was upset about it and wished that they had more of a drive, then I would say let them take the medication if they want to. If it would help them, then that's great." At least implicitly, my interviewees accepted the possibility that the availability of medical approaches to sexual disinterest might prevent people from coming to identify as asexual. Some explicitly acknowledged and accepted the fact that the availability of medical approaches to sexual disinterest might lead people who had previously identified as asexual to give up that label and leave the asexual community.

A few of my interviewees went even further than accepting movement between the labels of HSDD and asexuality, actually allowing for people to identify as asexual while pursuing medical approaches to sexual disinterest. Four of my interviewees said that although they identified as asexual, they would consider using a medical intervention in the future to increase their level of sexual interest, if an effective intervention were to be developed. These interviewees did not see this interest as necessarily in conflict with their identity as asexual. As one interviewee stated, "It's kind of like where if you identify as a lesbian but if you date a guy, then it's like, 'Oh, you're not a real lesbian.' Well, that's bullshit because I'm still me—behaviors and identity are not ever congruent—they're not ever 100 percent congruent." This interviewee, in particular, expressed the idea that even if she actively worked to increase her level of sexual desire, she could still identify as asexual and participate in asexual communities if doing so continued to feel appropriate to her.

I argue that asexual activists and the self-identified asexual individuals I spoke to were in the process of articulating something like a queer feminist approach to HSDD. They combined a critique of the assumptions underlying the definition of HSDD and of the normalizing power of HSDD with a tolerance for medical approaches to sexual disinterest. At the same time, in allowing for movement between the categories of asexuality and HSDD, or even allowing for someone to claim an asexual identity while seeking treatment for sexual disinterest, these activists and the individuals I spoke to avoided essentializing either asexuality or HSDD. Not surprisingly, the individuals I spoke to sometimes adopted the neoliberal language of "choice" to justify their tolerance for medical approaches to sexual disinterest (in other words, they argued that people should have the "choice" to pursue medical treatments if they wanted to); however, because this neoliberal language of choice was coupled with a critique of the pathologization of sexual disinterest, they avoided a complete endorsement of the tenets of neoliberalism.

A Queer Feminist Approach to Sexuopharmaceuticals

I end this chapter where I started—conflicted, in regards to both Viagra and to Addyi. Clearly, these types of interventions are designed to facilitate normative forms of sexuality—in the case of Viagra, penile-vaginal sexuality and, in the case of Addyi, female willingness to engage in sexual activities with male partners. As discursive formations, they potentially strengthen the social incitement of phallocentric desires and activities, likely at the expense of other (already marginalized) sexual possibilities. In addition, they do little to solve, and may very well be making more tolerable, social problems such as sexual violence, sexual inequality, and a lack of sexual and reproductive health education and services.

And yet, Viagra has been used in demonstrably queer ways, and Addyi may well be "queered" as well. In addition, even when used in normative ways, Viagra and Addyi may well enhance the sexual satisfaction of individuals. And, particularly in a society that has not been designed to promote sexual flourishing, pharmaceutical treatments may actually be the only intervention that works for some people.

Given these contradictions, themselves the product of our deeply unjust society, my compromised position has been to focus my activism not on opposing (or supporting) sexuopharmaceuticals but on changing the broader structures that play a role in creating sexual dissatisfaction, while working to achieve sexual and gender justice. Feminist activists and scholars can focus our attention on projects of sexual justice: advocating for comprehensive sexual education and sexual health and reproductive services, working to end sexual violence, fighting for the rights of sexual minorities, challenging racist sexual stereotypes, and more. We also certainly do need to put guidelines in place to ensure that these drugs are not directly forced on anyone and are not used in an obviously abusive manner, for example, by requiring physicians prescribing sexuopharmaceuticals to first screen patients for intimate partner violence (although, see Lavis et al. 2005). In addition, we can put guidelines in place that can temper some of the normative impulses of sexuopharmaceuticals as a discursive formation, such as requiring physicians prescribing sexuopharmaceuticals to first provide patients with information about asexual identities (a point I return to in the Conclusion). However, I think we should also allow individuals, in consultation with their communities, to decide to use these drugs if they think doing so will increase their sexual satisfaction and allow them to lead more fulfilling lives. My expectation is that as society becomes more sexually just, sexual dissatisfaction and the desire to address sexual dissatisfaction through medical intervention will decrease, although neither may ever disappear entirely. At the same time, my expectation is that as society becomes more sexually just, sexuopharmaceuticals will be used in ever more creative, playful, divergent, and queer ways.

CHAPTER 5

Constructing Fat, Constructing Fat Stigma

RETHINKING WEIGHT-REDUCTION INTERVENTIONS

As Susie Orbach so famously stated, fat is a feminist issue (Orbach 1997). Contemporary sexist and Eurocentric appearance norms that equate feminine beauty with extreme thinness have caused women untold pain and suffering. Weight-loss interventions, from diet programs that focus on calorie counting and physical activity to bariatric surgeries that aim to alter the size of the stomach and intestines, have long been the subject of feminist critique and censure. If I were ranking medical interventions involving gender norms from those provoking in me (and probably in many feminists) the least initial suspicion to the most initial suspicion, weight-loss interventions would certainly fall at or near the end of the list along with breast-enlargement surgeries and related "cosmetic" procedures. However, in this chapter, I will argue that even in the case of "extreme" weight-loss interventions such as bariatric surgeries, the political and ethical considerations involved are thorny and contradictory, and it may be prudent to focus, once again, on addressing larger structural issues while recognizing that some individuals can use bariatric surgery as a pathway to flourishing.

The issue of weight-loss interventions differs from transition-related interventions and sexuopharmaceutical interventions, in part because of the scope of the weight-loss industry and, more critically, because unlike in the other two cases, in recent years, weight-loss promotion has been explicitly approached from a public health and policy perspective—in other words, from a population-level and not just an individual-level perspective.[1] While many public health approaches to weight are roughly equivalent to traditional biomedical interventions in terms of their logic, there is also a subset of public health approaches ("critical public health" and/or public health focused on the "social determinants of health") that offers both a different analysis and a different set of recommendations. Part of my argument in this chapter is that critical public health approaches to weight do complicate some feminist/fat-positive positions on weight (and vice versa) and that combining the best of feminist/fat-positive perspectives on weight with the best of critical public health perspectives on weight leads to a more nuanced but still critical position on weight-loss interventions like bariatric surgery.

Before turning to the broader argument of the chapter, I begin with a brief analysis of First Lady Michelle Obama's "Let's Move" campaign, an effort by Obama to address childhood obesity in the United States. Obama's campaign was censured by critics on the right and the left. While critiques from the right clearly reflected bias against "big government," I also argue that in their failure to combine feminist/fat-positive and critical public health approaches, leftist critics were unable to offer a totally adequate reading of both the politically conservative and politically radical aspects of the campaign. This case demonstrates the importance of combining these two approaches in order to more fully understand the ethical, political, and social effects of weight-loss interventions.

I then turn to an analysis of traditional feminist/fat-positive and then critical public health approaches to weight and fatness. Both approaches offer powerful insights into the social and cultural construction of weight and fatness, but each approach on its own can miss key aspects of the picture. Feminist approaches to fatness are useful for their critique of our cultural obsession with thinness and weight loss (and the consequences of this obsession for women in particular) and for the ways in which they challenge stigma against fat people and work to revalue fatness. However, feminist approaches can miss the ways in which fatness is produced, in part, by public policies and corporate decisions that differentially burden women, people of color, and low-income people. Critical public health approaches to weight are useful precisely for their focus on the "social determinants" of weight. However, even critical public health approaches are flawed when they heighten social pressure to be thin and/or increase stigma against fat people. Thus, I argue that combining the best elements of these approaches leads to a more complete understanding of weight and fat as political and social issues.

I finally turn to addressing what this combined perspective suggests in terms of medical and surgical interventions to promote weight loss, with a focus on bariatric surgeries. Here I argue that medical and surgical interventions to promote weight loss do not address and may even exacerbate the structural issues that lead to both fat-related stigma and the differential production of fatness; however, these interventions still may be a survival strategy in a unjust world and, compared to other individualistic interventions such as diet and exercise, may actually have some advantages from a feminist perspective.

A brief note about terminology: I use the terms "fat" and "weight," but not "obese" or "overweight," unless I am quoting literature that uses the latter terms. The term "fat" is used by many fat-positive scholars and activists in an effort to reclaim the word and combat stigma. I do not use "obese" or "overweight" because they connote disease to many and are perceived by many fat people to carry stigma (Wann 2009).

MICHELLE OBAMA AND "LET'S MOVE"

It has been common for first ladies to pick a cause to champion during their husband's tenure in office. Claudia "Lady Bird" Johnson championed neighborhood "beautification," Nancy Reagan told the public to "Just Say No" to drugs, Hilary Clinton took on healthcare reform, and Laura Bush encouraged literacy. In 2010, First Lady Michelle Obama announced her ambitious "Let's Move" campaign, intended to "solve the problem of childhood obesity." Primarily focused on encouraging children to engage in more physical activity and on making "healthy" food more available in schools, the campaign also included celebrity endorsers, the creation of a kitchen garden at the White House, and numerous public appearances by the first lady (including an appearance on the weight-loss reality show *The Biggest Loser*), among other initiatives (Grey 2016; Obama 2012; Tanne 2010).

While praised by many in public health and medicine, Obama and her campaign faced criticism from both the left and the right. Some of the radical potential of the campaign was recognized by those on the right, who objected to the so-called big government approach taken by Obama. Critics on the right complained that Obama and the government were trying to dictate children's diets, thereby undermining parental authority (Oliphant 2011). The challenge Obama posed to the U.S. racial order was clearly recognized by these critics—Obama, as a black woman, was daring to suggest that she knew better than white parents what was best for white children, thereby challenging historically entrenched ideas about the inferiority of black mothering (D. E. Roberts 1993, 1999). The libertarian commitment to small government and the racial order was restored when Donald Trump became president in 2016 and his administration began to roll back nutrition standards for school cafeterias (Jacobs 2018).

While the right, in their outrage, seemed to recognize the more transgressive aspects of the campaign (while recognizing none of the actual problems), many on the left seemed to largely ignore the campaign—there was little left scholarly or activist commentary on the campaign outside of fat-positive activist spaces. Still, there were many fat-positive activists who challenged Obama's focus on weight rather than health and expressed concern that the campaign would increase the stigmatization and bullying of fat children (Association for Size Diversity and Health 2010; Macsta 2010). In an interview about the campaign, fat-positive activist Marilyn Warring stated, "The Let's Move campaign has this goal of 'solving the childhood obesity epidemic within one generation.' That's a terrible goal . . . basically what they are saying is we don't like fat children in our society, we don't want there to be any fat children" (Jonassen 2011).[2] These activist and academic critiques adequately captured some of the problems inherent in Obama's approach but also missed some of the radical potential of her approach.

In one of the few feminist academic analyses of the campaign, scholar Brittany Cooper identifies both conservative and transgressive aspects of the campaign but still fails to capture the full picture. Cooper does place Obama's self-presentation within a long tradition of black female respectability politics and recognizes the class politics of Obama's health campaign, writing,

> [Obama's] commitment to healthy food choices and regular exercise for children has become a central cause during her first years in the White House. In this regard, Obama's muscular arms signal very different possibilities for black women than those signaled by Sojourner Truth's muscular arms. Truth's arms were muscular because of the back breaking labor she was forced to do; Obama's arms are muscular, because she has the familial and professional support to build exercise into her daily schedule ... Obama's muscular arms symbolize her economic capacity to prioritize herself and her health and her access to the privileges of work/life balance. (B. Cooper 2010, 53)

And yet, for Cooper, the fact that Obama is a black woman makes her presentation of her own toned body and her Let's Move campaign politically transgressive. On Obama's refusal to stop wearing sleeveless dresses and short pants, she writes,

> This nonvocal, insistent self-assertion is a direct challenge to the politics of respectability ... Obama uses the public's fascination with her physique to champion healthy lifestyles, work/life balance for families (particularly for mothers), and better eating habits for children in a nation fast approaching a childhood obesity epidemic. This deft reappropriation of a potentially limiting and damaging public discourse about her body is a prime example of the ways black women use embodied discourse to transform not only public perceptions of themselves but the lives of citizens more generally. (B. Cooper 2010, 54)

For Cooper, then, the class and respectability politics embodied in Obama's campaign are subject to critique, but Obama's resistance to white supremacy renders other problems with her campaign invisible—for Cooper, Obama's focus on reducing "childhood obesity" is not subject for concern.

It is my contention that critics from the right actually recognized some of what was positive about the campaign—public health-inspired system-level interventions that sought to make "healthy" food and opportunities for physical activity more accessible, all helmed by a black woman. At the same time, critics from the left identified real problems with the campaign—its potential for increasing stigma against fatness—while ignoring the more radical aspects of the campaign. Cooper succeeds in identifying the class conservatism of the campaign, while also recognizing Obama's challenge to the racial order, but fails to acknowledge the sizeism of the campaign. In their failure to combine feminist/ fat-positive approaches to weight with critical public health approaches to weight, none of the critics from the left offered a wholly adequate analysis of the Let's Move campaign. In the rest of the chapter, I hope to demonstrate that only by combining intersectional feminist and fat-positive approaches to weight with critical public health approaches to weight are we able to see both what was "right" and what was "wrong" with Obama's approach, while also envisioning more politically progressive alternatives.

Context: The So-Called Obesity Epidemic

For the past two decades, in the United States and globally, there has been significant attention paid to the so-called obesity epidemic by medical practitioners, public health officials, politicians, and the media. According to those who are concerned about "obesity," rates of fatness are rising rapidly, which should provoke widespread alarm. According to these analysts, obesity negatively impacts the health of a country, as weight is correlated with health conditions, including heart disease, stroke, type 2 diabetes, and certain types of cancer. In addition, according to these analysts, fat costs a society dearly in terms of medical expenses and lost productivity (Centers for Disease Control and Prevention [CDC] 2007). In recent years, government and public health officials, medical professionals and researchers, the media, and the diet and weight-loss industry have come together to wage a so-called war on obesity (Herndon 2002).

Feminist, Queer, and Disability Studies Approaches to Fat

Feminist scholars have made key contributions to our understanding of the social and cultural construction of weight and fatness. According to feminist scholars and activists, including Susan Bordo and Jean Kilbourne, Western society's obsession with female thinness regulates the behavior of all women (fat, thin, and in between). Women and girls spend enormous amounts of time, energy, and resources trying to be thin and to take up less space. This quest for thinness saps the power of women and girls and has enormous consequences such as psychological distress and disordered eating (Bordo 2004; Kilbourne 2004). In a classic argument, Bordo suggests that eating disorders are only the extreme of a spectrum of eating-disordered behavior in women that is caused by Western society's cultural valuation of female slimness (Bordo 2004). In fact, Bordo questions the definitions of anorexia and bulimia as "pathological states," arguing that women with anorexia or bulimia accurately perceive the real cultural benefits of slimness and the cultural costs of fatness. In addition, according to a number of scholars, the weight-loss industry and the beauty industry fan the flames of this cultural obsession with thinness in order to increase profits (while other industries simultaneously promote overconsumption) (Lyons 2009; Featherstone 2007; N. Wolf 2002).

At the same time, feminists within the field of fat studies have demonstrated that fat people (and especially fat women) are subject to bias, discrimination, stigma, and abuse. According to these scholars, fat people are often portrayed as lazy, immoral, and/or unintelligent, and they are viewed as objects of pity, ridicule, or disgust. In addition, according to feminist critics, the built environment, from school desks to airplane seats, is not designed to accommodate people of size (Wann 2009).

Feminist critics have also questioned our society's equation of fat with ill health. As Annemarie Jutel argues, the current focus on fat is really about appearance but is shrouded in the language of health in order to secure legitimacy (Jutel 2001, 2005). Paul Campos argues that the labeling of fat as unhealthy legitimizes white middle-class prejudices against poor people and people of color (Campos 2004). Analysts have critiqued the use of body mass index (BMI) as a measure of fat/health (Nicholls 2013) and have argued that the association between fat and ill health is mostly correlational, not causational (Burgard 2009); that fat people can be healthy and thin people can be unhealthy (Burgard 2009); and that "moderate" heaviness may actually confer protective health benefits in some cases (Ernsberger 2009). Careful reviews of the available data suggest that only at extreme ends of the spectrum (very fat or very thin) is weight related to longevity and that "moderate" heaviness may actually be correlated with a longer life span (Bacon and Aphramor 2011). In addition, while fatness is correlated with an increased risk for many diseases, these diseases may be caused by other factors, such as nutrient intake, levels of physical activity, or socioeconomic status, that also covary with weight (Bacon and Aphramor 2011).

In addition, feminist critics have argued that some or many of the negative health consequences of fat may actually be the result not of fat itself but of stigma and discrimination against fat people (Ernsberger 2009). Stigma and discrimination may produce ill health through a number of pathways. For example, fat people are discriminated against in education and employment, which can increase economic insecurity, and economic insecurity is related to poorer health outcomes (R. M. Puhl, Andreyeva, and Brownell 2008; Roehling, Roehling, and Pichler 2007; Ernsberger 2009; R. Puhl and Brownell 2001). In addition, fat people are discriminated against by healthcare professionals, which means that fat people may avoid going to the doctor and/or may receive inadequate healthcare when they do go to the doctor (R. Puhl and Brownell 2001; Amy et al. 2005). Finally, researchers have found that perceived discrimination and stigma increase stress, which can produce negative health outcomes (Meyer 2003; Pascoe and Smart Richman 2009). Because stigma and discrimination are connected to poor health outcomes, to the extent that antiobesity campaigns like Michelle Obama's "Let's Move" campaign contribute to stigma against fat people, they may actually do more harm than good (Bacon and Aphramor 2011; Burgard 2009).

Feminist scholars have also argued that very few people who attempt to lose weight are actually successful at doing so long term (Gaesser 2009; Burgard 2009) and that repeatedly losing and regaining weight (also known as "yo-yo dieting" or "weight cycling") can have negative health consequences (Burgard 2009; Bacon and Aphramor 2011). For example, there is some evidence to suggest that hypertension (commonly thought to be the result of weight) is actually caused by the stress of weight cycling (Bacon and Aphramor 2011). In addition, according to critics, there is not enough evidence to conclude that weight loss (even if maintained) actually improves health outcomes, and there is some evidence to suggest that weight loss might actually negatively impact health (Bacon and Aphramor 2011).

Finally, and more broadly, disability studies scholars have questioned our society's obsession with health and our equation of health with moral goodness (Metzl and Kirkland 2010). In the case of weight, Western society clearly associates thinness with both health and moral goodness and fatness with both ill health and moral failing (especially laziness and a lack of self-control), while elevating the pursuit of health (and thus thinness) over all other goals. In this moral universe, allowing oneself to be fat (or even embracing fatness) because one prioritizes other goals—such as the pleasures of eating or repose—becomes simply unimaginable.[3]

FEMINIST AND FAT-POSITIVE INTERVENTIONS

Over the past forty years, feminist and fat studies activists and scholars have launched a number of campaigns to transform the way our society approaches weight and fatness. "Love Your Body" campaigns have encouraged all women to embrace their bodies and to reject our society's obsession with evaluating women based on how closely they approximate white female beauty ideals.[4] In addition, feminists have called out the fashion, advertising, and magazine industries, in particular, for featuring incredibly slim models and actresses and for altering photographs of women to make them appear thinner, bustier, and/or whiter.[5] Campaigns that simply tell women to love their bodies are unlikely to be effective in a culture that so heavily values female slimness, whiteness, and "beauty," but campaigns that work to change broader structures (such as creating new regulations for advertisements) may have a greater effect.

In a connected but somewhat different vein, Fat Acceptance, Fat Pride, and Fat Liberation efforts have specifically worked to decrease stigma against fatness, to encourage fat people to embrace their fatness and claim fatness as a political identity, and to represent fatness as valuable, desirable, and/or sexy (Wann 2009;

McAllister 2009; Burgard et al. 2009; C. Cooper 2010). The Fat Acceptance/Pride/ Liberation movement has a long history; for example, the National Association to Advance Fat Acceptance (NAAFA) was founded in 1969 to protect the rights and improve the quality of life of fat people ("The National Association to Advance Fat Acceptance" n.d.), and in 1973, members of the Fat Underground, a Los Angeles–based organization, wrote the "Fat Liberation Manifesto" demanding rights for fat people and identifying the diet industry as the enemy (S. Fishman 1998). In recent years, the Fat Acceptance/Pride/Liberation movement has established a strong online presence.[6]

More recently, the Health at Every Size (HAES) movement has attempted to move the healthcare field away from its focus on weight loss. Growing out of the efforts of both healthcare professionals and fat acceptance activists, the HAES movement still uses the language of "health," but instead of focusing on weight per se, adherents encourage first, bodily acceptance and respect for bodily diversity; second, learning to eat based on internal cues of hunger and satiety; and, third, finding joy in moving one's body and active embodiment (Burgard 2009; Bacon and Aphramor 2011). Supporters also claim that women who participate in support groups or "intervention" groups that use the HAES approach show improvements in physiological measures (e.g., blood pressure), health behaviors (e.g., levels of physical activity), and psychosocial outcomes (e.g., body satisfaction) (Bacon and Aphramor 2011), but the evidence here appears to be mixed or incomplete (Provencher et al. 2007; Leblanc et al. 2012; Provencher et al. 2009; Penney and Kirk 2015).[7] The movement's focus on respect for bodily diversity and on promoting "healthy" behaviors as opposed to weight loss is certainly very helpful in a fat-phobic society. In addition, the fact that the HAES approach continues to use the language of health and to focus, in its own way, on promoting health may make the HAES message more palatable to skeptical health professionals than the Fat Liberation message, and thus, the HAES movement could be thought of as a harm reduction strategy, designed to temper the worst aspects of current medical approaches to weight. Still, even with this seemingly more moderate message, the HAES movement has been criticized by some in the medical profession (Worth 2010; Sainsbury and Hay 2014).

In addition, some feminists, disability rights activists, and Fat Liberation activists have criticized the HAES movement. Echoing the approach of feminist science studies scholars, Deborah Lupton critiques the movement for naturalizing the notion of "internal cues," arguing that internal cues are inevitably the product of an admixture of biology, society, and individual life history.[8] In addition, Lupton questions whether a message about bodily acceptance can really be effective in a society that discriminates against fat people (Lupton 2012). Welsh argues that the HAES framework still promotes healthism, or the belief that individuals should strive to be healthy and that (fat) bodies are only acceptable to the extent that they are healthy bodies (Welsh 2011). Disability activists have argued that this leaves "unhealthy" fat people and/or fat people with disabilities in a stigmatized space (S. E. Smith 2014). The notion of "joyful" physical activity should also be problematized—it is entirely conceivable that for some or even many people, the level of physical activity required to actually improve "health" (if this is what one desires) may never be experienced as "joyful."[9] The HAES movement's message may be pollyannaish—suggesting that health can be achieved joyfully and without sacrifice. In general, while recognizing the influence of structural forces on the ability of individuals to eat according to internal cues and engage in "joyful" physical activity, the HAES framework focuses on individual behavior change rather than structural solutions and thus, on its own, is incomplete from a feminist perspective.

LIMITATIONS OF FEMINIST APPROACHES

In sum, feminist approaches to weight are useful for their critique of our cultural obsession with thinness (and the consequences of this obsession for women in particular) and for the ways in which they challenge stigma against fat people and work to revalue fatness. However, as discussed by fat studies scholar Kathleen LeBesco, these approaches can be problematically essentialist when scholars or activists argue that some people are simply born fat and that fatness is an unalterable property of the body (LeBesco 2004, 2009a). Feminist science studies scholars have critiqued activist efforts to essentialize sexual orientation (see, e.g., Terry 1999). As in the case of gay and lesbian activists and sexual orientation, there are good reasons for fat activists to argue that fat is genetically determined— if fat is seen as genetically determined, this could (1) decrease stigma against fat people because society would no longer view fat people as (morally) responsible for their fatness and (2) protect fat people from pressure to engage in weight-loss interventions as it would be clear that these interventions could not achieve their goal. However, it is also possible (as in the case of sexual orientation) that efforts to locate a "fat gene" could also lead to efforts to eliminate fat people through procedures such as preimplantation genetic diagnosis (PGD) and/or prenatal testing followed by abortion. In addition, although understandable, these kinds of essentialist arguments can be a problem for progressive projects, as progressive projects often seek to replace a commonplace attribution of observed differences to unchanging biological roots with an understanding of these differences as produced by social inequalities and as subject to transformation (Phillips 2010).[10] At the same time, these kinds of arguments do not protect those people whose (fat) bodies and/or (queer) desires are fluid, clearly chosen, or do not seem to be the result of genetic causes (at least not in any straightforward way).

In addition, as LeBesco also notes, many traditional feminist and fat studies approaches to weight have understandably attempted to deny any connection between weight and health, thus potentially losing the ability to acknowledge some fatness as "healthy" and some fatness as "unhealthy." LeBesco asks, "How can fat people own their own realities—that sometimes fat is healthy and sometimes it isn't—and still keep their political agenda intact?" (LeBesco 2009a, 153). In addition to potentially flattening out nuances, refusing any connection between weight and health may indeed challenge negative perceptions of fat people, but it does not fundamentally challenge generalized stigma against illness and, to the extent that it represents an attempt to create distance between fatness and disability-related stigma, this move may make it more difficult to form coalitions between fat liberation movements and disability liberation movements (see also LeBesco 2015; Herndon 2002). Perhaps more important, many feminist fat studies approaches do not offer many resources for addressing the ways in which fatness may be produced, in part, by public policies and corporate decisions that differentially affect people of color and low-income people.[11]

CRITICAL PUBLIC HEALTH, ENVIRONMENTAL JUSTICE, AND FOOD SYSTEMS APPROACHES TO FAT

While feminist and fat studies approaches have critiqued our society's obsession with slimness and weight loss and have called out the diet, exercise, and fashion industries for reinforcing or even creating this obsession in order to increase profits, critical public health, environmental justice, and food-systems scholars have argued that an individual's size and weight are very much influenced by their social and physical environment, including the food they have access to, what type of work they do, whether they have space or time for physical recreation, how much they are able to sleep, whether and to what extent they experience stress, and whether they are exposed to environmental toxins (Prince 2009). This social and physical environment is influenced by corporate decisions and public policies (everything from agricultural policy, taxation policy, zoning regulations, communication policy, urban planning, transportation policy, food subsidy policies, and trade policies) (Kaestner 2009; M. Nestle and Jacobson 2000; American Public Health Association [APHA] 2007; R. P. Lopez and Hynes 2006). In terms of corporate decisions, the food industry benefits from marketing and selling calorie-rich foods and drinks that contain high levels of saturated and trans fats, added sugars, and/or sodium (which I will refer to here as "less-nutritious food" for purposes of brevity) (M. Nestle and Jacobson 2000; M. Nestle 2013).[12] To date, our public policy choices have largely served to create an environment in which people have more access to less-nutritious food than to more-nutritious food and often have little time or opportunity for physical activity (Kaestner 2009; M. Nestle and Jacobson 2000; APHA 2007; R. P. Lopez and Hynes 2006). It is also worth noting here that, as ethicists and food systems analysts have pointed out, our current food production system fosters environmental destruction, cruelty to nonhuman animals, and the exploitation of human agribusiness workers both in the United States and in "Global South" countries (APHA 2007; Guthman 2011). In any case, to the extent that access to less-nutritious food and a lack of access to opportunities or time for physical activity are "unhealthy," corporate and public policy choices have contributed to the production of ill health. Incidentally or not, to the extent that less-nutritious food and a lack of access to opportunities or time for physical activity are tied to weight gain, corporate and public policy choices have contributed to the production of fat people.

Importantly, critical public health, environmental justice, and food-systems scholars have pointed out that corporate decisions and public policies differentially burden certain communities. Low-income communities and communities of color are those that have the least access to more-nutritious food and the resources and time required for physical activity, and they may also face disproportionate exposure to environmental causes of weight gain. For example, according to a 2013 article published in the *Journal of the Academy of Nutrition and Dietetics*, for adults, diet quality generally improved with income level (with the exception of sodium), although low-income children actually had better diet quality than higher-income children, which was thought to reflect their greater participation in food-assistance programs (Hiza et al. 2013). As another example, according to a 2006 article published in *Pediatrics*, neighborhoods (specifically census block groups) with lower socioeconomic status (SES) had fewer recreational facilities, and adolescents living in these neighborhoods reported lower levels of moderate to vigorous physical activity (Gordon-Larsen et al. 2006). Other factors tied to weight gain—such as stress and exposure to environmental toxins, also differentially impact low-income communities and communities of color (Adler and Newman 2002). Studies have also found that food insecurity is correlated with weight gain (Finney Rutten et al. 2012).

In part as a result of these disparities, in the United States, fat is differentially distributed by gender, race/ethnicity, socioeconomic status, and residential location. According to a nationally representative data set, on average, women are more likely to be fat than men, African Americans are more likely to be fat than whites, and African American women in particular have comparatively high rates of fatness.[13] The same nationally representative data set shows that populations with lower SES have higher rates of fatness than populations with higher SES, although, interestingly, this is most true for white women, and the relationship between SES and fat is complex and has become less clear in recent prevalence trends (Kumanyika et al. 2008). Rates of fatness also vary by region; states in the South generally have higher rates of fatness than states in the North and West. Also of note is the fact that rural areas tend to have higher rates of fatness than suburban and urban areas (Kumanyika et al. 2008).

Although less often remarked on by critical public health scholars, access to more-nutritious food and opportunities and time for physical activity are also indirectly influenced by the intersection of gender and racial politics (in addition to the direct relationship between the marginalization of women and people of color and higher rates of fatness among women and people of color than among men and white people). For example, some critical public health scholars have identified the rise of urban sprawl and the suburbanization of the United States as one factor that has contributed to increasing rates of fatness (e.g., R. Lopez 2004). At the same time, using an intersectional approach, gender scholars have argued that the state, urban planners, developers, and architects designed post–World War II suburban neighborhoods based on a racialized, sexualized, and gendered notion of "separate spheres"—namely the idea that middle-class white women will occupy the private space of the home (a site of consumption and reproduction) while middle-class white men will occupy the public space of the workplace (a site of production) (e.g., England 1993). At the same time, postwar suburbanization in the United States was tied to "white flight"—namely, the movement of whites out of cities as blacks moved into urban areas, which became, in turn, centers of poverty that lacked grocery stores and safe sites for physical recreation (e.g., Crowder 2000). Thus, it can be argued that the very architecture that contributes to fatness reflects and reinforces the intersection of patriarchal and racist norms. At the same time, women of all races often remain responsible for their family's food consumption and health-related activities (like exercise) even when they participate in the paid workforce (the so-called second shift, or the unpaid reproductive labor done by people, especially women, who also participate in the paid labor force) (Hochschild and Machung 2012). Thus, women who are overburdened by work and family responsibilities and/or women resisting traditional feminine roles may, for example, turn to quick and convenient sources of food that are less nutritious ("fast food"). As sociologists Sarah Bowen, Sinikka Elliott, and Joslyn Brenton argue, as a result of time pressures, trade-offs to save money, and unappreciative family members, women often find home cooking to be a burden and turn to commercially prepared food as a better alternative (Bowen, Elliott, and Brenton 2014). Thus, it can be argued that a lack of social support for caregiving and gender ideologies that disproportionately burden women with caregiving responsibilities also contribute to increasing rates of fatness.

Critical Public Health Interventions

Based on these insights, I would argue that we cannot simply ignore the factors that have contributed to poor nutrition and a lack of physical activity as these factors have disproportionately burdened low-income people and people of color and contributed to environmental degradation while also reflecting and reinforcing troubling gender and racial norms. I am interested in critical public health approaches that seek to alter the world so that people, regardless of income or neighborhood of residence, have easy access to good-tasting, nutritious food and plenty of opportunities for recreation and physical activity and are less exposed to the environmental factors that lead to weight gain. These interventions include improving public transportation; installing sidewalks, bike paths, and greenspaces; making playgrounds more accessible to different body types; improving food labeling; subsidizing more-nutritious food, especially in schools; eliminating current subsidies for less-nutritious food; eliminating or at least reducing the environmental toxins that may be contributing to weight gain; and improving social safety nets in order to reduce stress, to name a few (Nestle and Jacobsen 2000; Kaestner 2009; Kumanyika et al. 2008). Michelle Obama's "Let's Move" campaign focused on some of these interventions, such as increasing access to more-nutritious food in schools, but paid less attention to others, such as reducing environmental toxins.

Limitations of Public Health Approaches

However, I want to make it clear here that I most certainly do not endorse many public health approaches to weight or many of the so-called solutions that have been proposed to the "problem" of fatness. In general, the entire effort to characterize "obesity" as an epidemic is deeply problematic. J. Eric Oliver critiques William Dietz of the CDC for creating a series of maps in the late 1990s that seemed to depict "obesity" as an infectious disease, increasing in prevalence over time and "spreading" from one state to another. Oliver argues that it was primarily these maps that led doctors, public health officials, the media, and, eventually, the American public to conceptualize "obesity" as an "epidemic" (Oliver 2006). And the very conceptualization of obesity as an epidemic has led to panic, stigma, and pressure to adopt unwanted and/or ineffective weight-loss interventions.

In my estimation, we should be critical of all "individualist" public health solutions to weight as well as "structuralist" solutions that present an overly simplified picture of the connection between weight and health and encourage moral panic about the so-called obesity epidemic.[14] In addition, even the approaches that I endorsed above are limited and potentially damaging on their own unless combined with feminist and disability studies approaches.

By individualist public health approaches, I mean those approaches that involve the state or civil society in seeking to identify "overweight" or "obese" individuals and encouraging or forcing them to lose weight through dieting and exercise. Feminists have long been critical of these types of interventions (behavioral change through health promotion campaigns) as they tend to focus on individual behavior change to the exclusion of broader structural changes (Daykin and Naidoo 1995). These types of approaches are particularly problematic when it comes to weight, because they contribute to stigma against fat people by assigning moral responsibility for fatness (read as ill health) and for weight loss (read as health) to the individual. A particularly egregious example of this type of public health approach can be seen in the widely criticized campaign run by Children's Healthcare of Atlanta in which print and TV ads showed images of actual overweight children, such as a billboard picturing a fat girl with the tagline "It's hard to be a little girl if you're not" (Lohr n.d.). In her work, LeBesco identifies as particularly pernicious such state efforts to combat "obesity" as BMI "report card" bills—laws requiring public schools to weigh children and notify parents if their children are "at risk" of "obesity"—and state efforts, in some cases, to curtail the custody rights of the parents of overweight children (LeBesco 2011).

In her book, *Weighing In: Obesity, Food Justice, and the Limits of Capitalism*, Julie Guthman argues that many seemingly more benign solutions to the "obesity epidemic"—such as efforts to encourage the consumption of "local" and "organic" food—are individualistic solutions that are primarily pursuable by middle- and upper-class consumers (as exemplified in Michelle Obama's creation of a kitchen garden at the White House). In addition, these types of "solutions" do not fundamentally alter the broader food system, which encourages the production and consumption of cheap, less-nutritious food, and also ignore other causes of "obesity" such as environmental toxins (Guthman 2011). At the same time, as suggested by the discussion above, "solutions" such as encouraging people to eat local and organic food (and the demonization of "fast food") may especially burden women if they remain disproportionately responsible for food preparation. Kim Hall also points out that the food justice and alternative food movements often rely on a "metaphysics of purity"—in which "real" food can be distinguished from "artificial" food—and on "alimentary ableism"—in which "real" food is desirable because it prevents or cures disability. In addition, as Hall suggests, these movements often romanticize the past, relying heavily on a sexist and racist imagining of the past in which yeomen (white, male) farmers raised their own food that was then "home cooked" and served by their wives. In the article, Hall also introduces the perspective of Catherine Kudlick, a blind disability studies scholar. For Kudlick, having autonomy over her food choices was sometimes more important than nutritional content in determining the worth of her food (Hall 2015). From Kudlick's perspective, I believe we can derive the more general claim that what makes a particular food "good" depends on more than its nutritional content and whether it is produced sustainably. Rather, what makes a particular eating pattern or food "good" or "healthy" must be determined based on the entire context of a person's life, in concert with a consideration of the myriad effects that producing and consuming this food will have on the human and nonhuman world.[15]

Although structural approaches are often better than individualistic approaches, even the approaches that focus on the "social determinants of size" can be deeply problematic. In her article, "The Environmental Account of Obesity: A Case for Feminist Skepticism," Anna Kirkland argues that so-called environmental approaches to fat can mask individualist and moralizing impulses. She notes that many efforts to change the so-called obesogenic environment really aim to alter the "choice architecture" of our society (a term not used by Kirkland but appropriate here)[16] such that the food and exercise choices of low-income and minority people more closely resemble the food and exercise choices of elites. Kirkland argues that many of the "liberals" advocating for these policies may have little or no understanding of the lived experiences of low-income people and people of color, and she posits that low-income people and people of color are already exerting agency in their food and exercise choices and that efforts to alter those choices run the risk of paternalism. In addition, she argues that environmental approaches can suggest that low-income people and people of color are victims of their environment in ways that elites are not. She also argues that, in practice, environmental approaches are likely to become punitive in nature. Finally, she makes the important point that "we" (by which she means elite liberals) do not need the "excuse" of weight or even health to justify many of our goals, writing, "There are plenty of other reasons to promote public transit and farmer's markets, like sustainability, emissions control, and pleasure" (Kirkland 2011, 481).

In a similar vein, Anna Mollow argues that the "foodscape argument" (which Mollow also calls the "obesogenic environment" thesis and the "environmental theory of fatness") perpetuates fat phobia, racism, sexism, ableism, healthicism, and neoliberal values of personal responsibility while obscuring the problem of food poverty (Mollow 2016). She writes,

> After reflecting upon the above concerns, some progressive readers may be tempted to ask: what if we keep the foodscape argument but eliminate its politically problematic aspects? This is impossible, because the foodscape argument—which is premised on the notion that an entire group, fat people, is fundamentally not okay—is incompatible with progressive political ideals. Contending that fatness is caused by economic injustice, the foodscape argument imagines that an equitable world would be free of fatness and fat people. By contrast, a truly emancipatory approach to body diversity must work for a world that is free of fatphobia. (Mollow 2016, n.p.)

While I agree with both Kirkland and Mollow's critiques of structural approaches to fatness, I believe there are elements of these approaches that should, in fact, be combined with feminist, fat-positive, and disability-positive insights. Unlike Kirkland and Mollow, I think that structural approaches to weight should focus not just on food and exercise but also on other potential causes of weight gain, such as exposure to stress and environmental toxins. In addition, while the structural approach to weight recognizes that low-income people and people of color are disadvantaged by their lack of access to a broad range of foodscapes and physical activity–scapes and that marginalized groups often experience greater exposure to stressful events and environmental toxins, a structural approach to weight certainly does not suggest that dominant groups are not affected by their environments (as suggested by Mollow). In addition, I do not think that an environmental approach is necessarily founded on the premise that fat people, as an entire group, are "not ok" (as Mollow states and as Marilyn Warring stated in regards to Obama's Let's Move campaign), but rather that certain conditions (lack of opportunity for physical activity; lack of access to affordable, convenient, tasty, and nutritious food; exposure to stress and environmental toxins; etc.) tend to promote weight gain, which can, in some cases, contribute to ill health, in a complex way. Still, it is absolutely the case that on their own, structural approaches to weight are limited and can promote stigma against fat people, and therefore, they must be combined with feminist, fat-positive, and disability-positive approaches that challenge fat phobia.

Combining the Best Elements of Different Approaches

As a result, I believe it is critical that we combine the best elements of feminist fat studies approaches with the best elements of critical public health approaches, while also taking into account insights from disability studies, food studies, and environmental studies. Feminist fat studies and critical public health have often been seen as antithetical to each other and sometimes see themselves as antithetical. In some ways, this is true—a feminist fat studies approach seeks to revalue and, indeed, "love" fatness, while a public health approach seeks to reduce the prevalence of fat in the future. However, my argument here is that they can and should be combined to produce the following plan of action for feminists: first, feminist scholars and activists must continue to call out our cultural obsession with thinness, particularly for women. In addition, we must continue to challenge stigma and discrimination against fat people. We must emphasize that many fat people are perfectly "healthy." At the same time, we must challenge the idea that there is a moral imperative to pursue health. We must affirm that other goals or pleasures (e.g., the pleasures of sugary foods or the pleasures of repose) might be more important than health for some people. Thus, we must affirm that even in cases where fat is "unhealthy," fatness and the pursuit of fatness may be perfectly congruent with and even necessary to an individual's overall flourishing.[17]

Second, we must continue to critique overly simplified claims about the connection between health and weight, and we must challenge punitive and individualist public health approaches to weight loss. At the same time, we should work to alter the broader structures of our society so that all who wish to eat more nutritious food and engage in physical activity have the opportunity to do so (and disability studies reminds us to make sure that opportunities for physical activity in particular are open to people with disabilities). We should also work to reduce other causes of weight gain, such as stress and environmental toxins. These changes will make it easier for those for whom fat is not conducive to a fulfilling life and who wish to lose weight (or avoid weight gain) to do so. At the same time, we must continue to insist that even if nutritious foods and opportunities for exercise are available, there is *no necessary moral obligation* to eat nutritious food or engage in physical activity.[18]

Finally, we must understand how our current global food systems impact food system workers, nonhuman animals, and the environment, and we must work to develop food systems that are sustainable; provide fair wages, benefits, and safe working conditions; and ensure the ethical treatment of food animals (APHA 2007). Had Michelle Obama's campaign dropped the language of obesity and even weight, and had she combined structural interventions to increase opportunities for physical activity and access to more-nutritious food with anti-bullying messages and programs designed to increase respect for bodily diversity, then the "Let's Move" campaign would have, in my estimation, better contributed to social justice.

In a society without fat phobia or discrimination against fat people, even if the environmental causes of fat are reduced and more nutritious food and opportunities for physical recreation are available to all, it is an open question whether there would be more or fewer fat people. The point of the approach I have outlined is not to produce a world without fatness (or thinness) but to produce a world where neither thinness nor fatness is socially imposed in unjust ways—whether through social norms that reward (and thus require) thinness or food deserts that leave certain neighborhoods without many food options.

What Then of Medical Weight-Loss Interventions?

Given this discussion, what are we to make of medical/surgical interventions designed to produce weight loss? Current biomedical approaches to weight loss include dieting, physical activity, behavior therapy, pharmacotherapy, and weight-loss surgery. As of the beginning of 2017, the Food and Drug Administration (FDA) in the United States had approved five prescription weight-loss drugs for long-term use: orlistat (Xenical) (also available over-the-counter as Alli) (originally approved in 1997), lorcaserin (Belviq) (2012), phentermine-topiramate (Qsymia) (2012), naltrexone-bupropion (Contrave) (2014), and liraglutide (Saxenda) (2014). Xenical reduces intestinal absorption of fats into the body; Belviq, Qsymia, and Contrave act on the brain (likely to reduce appetite); and Saxenda (originally approved to treat diabetes) is an analogue of a satiety-signaling intestinal hormone (and is administered through a once-a-day injection). Other weight-loss drugs—most notoriously fenfluramine and dexfenfluramine

(Fen-Phen)—have been removed from the market due to associated health risks. Currently, weight-loss drugs are only recommended for people with a BMI ≥ 30 kg/m² or a BMI ≥ 27 kg/m² with "weight-related" health conditions. Reviews suggest that approved weight-loss medications increase a person's chances of losing weight and lead to an average of 2.6 kg (5.7 lbs.) to 8.8 kg (19.4 lbs.) of additional weight loss compared to placebo at one year, and there is some evidence that these drugs can reduce the chance that a person will develop type 2 diabetes. However, all of the drugs have side effects and risks, and there are little data about whether the drugs lead to weight loss or improved health outcomes in the long term (Hiatt, Thomas, and Goldfine 2012; Khera et al. 2016; Colman 2005; Apovian et al. 2015; Padwal, Li, and Lau 2004).[19]

In addition to medication, surgery is also recommended as a "treatment" for overweight in some cases. In the United States, for adults, bariatric surgery is only recommended for patients with a BMI ≥ 40 kg/m² or a BMI ≥ 35 kg/m² with weight-related health conditions (or a BMI ≥ 30 kg/m² with weight-related health conditions for gastric banding only) ("Potential Candidates for Bariatric Surgery" n.d.). According to data from 2013, in the United States and Canada, the most commonly performed types of surgery are gastric sleeve (43 percent), gastric bypass (35.3 percent), and adjustable gastric banding (10 percent), with a small percentage of patients undergoing other forms of bariatric surgery. This represents a marked change from a decade ago, when adjustable gastric banding was by far the most commonly performed procedure (Angrisani et al. 2015).

In general, bariatric surgery works either by restricting the size of the stomach so people feel full sooner and eat less and/or by altering the small intestine in order to reduce the absorption of calories.[20] In gastric sleeve surgery, a significant portion of the stomach is removed and the remainder is shaped into a "tube" or "sleeve." In gastric bypass surgery, staples are used to create a small pouch in the upper part of the stomach and then the small intestine is cut from the bottom of the stomach and reattached to the newly created pouch, thus "bypassing" the lower part of the stomach. In gastric banding, a silicone band is placed around the stomach and tightened in order to make the stomach smaller. In the United States, bariatric surgery is almost always performed laparoscopically ("Types of Bariatric Surgery" n.d.). Reviews suggest that after two or more years, gastric bypass and gastric sleeve surgeries on average produce an "excess weight loss" (EWL)[21] of about 65 percent while gastric banding on average produces an "excess weight loss" of about 45 percent. Bariatric surgeries also can lead to remission or improvement in type 2 diabetes, hypertension, and hyperlipidemia (Puzziferri et al. 2014; Chang et al. 2014; Gloy et al. 2013).

There are significant side effects and risks associated with all bariatric surgeries. For gastric bypass, for example, immediate complications include leakage through staples or sutures, ulcers, blood clots, stretching of the pouch or esophagus, persistent vomiting and abdominal pain, inflammation of the gallbladder, and/or "failure" to lose weight, although all of these complications are rare or very rare. Nearly 30 percent of patients develop nutritional deficiencies, but these deficiencies can be avoided by taking supplements. More than one-third of patients develop gallstones, although, again, this can be avoided by taking supplements. Ten to 20 percent of patients require follow-up operations to correct complications, most commonly strictures and hernias. Death as a result of surgery or surgery-related complications is very rare. After surgery, patients must change their eating habits and are encouraged to eat small amounts and to chew their food well in order to avoid complications. Patients are also encouraged to become more physically active. Some patients elect to have "excess" skin removed via surgery. According to medical practitioners, bariatric surgery can have significant psychosocial effects, both positive and negative, including effects on relationships. Bariatric surgery seems to enjoy relatively high rates of patient satisfaction, and biomedical-oriented research suggests that bariatric surgery improves mental health, psychosocial status, and quality of life for the majority of patients, but also a significant minority of patients report no improvement in mental health or even a worsening of mental health after surgery (Brethauer, Chand, and Schauer 2006; "Bariatric Surgery Side Effects" n.d.; Ballantyne 2003; Müller et al. 2008; Karmali 2013). There is still insufficient evidence about the long-term effects of bariatric surgery (Puzziferri et al. 2014). In addition, there seems to be comparatively little clinical research into the effects of bariatric surgery on subjective well-being, suggesting that those approaching the issue from a biomedical perspective simply assume that weight loss leads to patient happiness.

The regressive aspects of medical and surgical weight-loss interventions should be clear based on what I have already written: these interventions are part of neoliberal body projects of normalization; they are pursued (despite their risks and side effects) primarily because of the stigmatization of fat bodies and panic around weight and health; in existing (and thus offering an "out"), they may pacify some fat people who would otherwise join body-positive and fat liberation movements; their very existence sends the message to fat people that society views their bodies as in need of correction; and they allow drug companies and bariatric surgeons to profit off of the social stigmatization of fatness.

Again, however, some critics of weight-loss interventions err in using discourses of naturalization to reject weight-loss surgeries. For example, in an otherwise incisive article criticizing the characterization of obesity as a disease, Oliver writes,

> Among general surgical procedures, bariatric surgery is unique in that it does not target a distressed or infected organ. Whereas all other general surgical procedures go after things such as an inflamed appendix or a sick gallbladder, bariatric surgeons target a healthy stomach and small intestine. Paradoxically,

> weight-loss doctors evaluate the various bariatric surgical procedures based on
> their capacity for creating 'mal-absorption,' the ability to make the stomach
> and small intestine dysfunctional. The Orwellian logic behind this process is
> telling: in order to 'cure' the imaginary 'disease' of obesity, doctors will surgi-
> cally alter a healthy organ and make it permanently sick to the point where it
> actually meets the technical definition of a disease. (Oliver 2006, 624–625)

Unfortunately, this kind of argument reinforces the idea that there are "actually" diseased organs, in contrast to the "imaginarily" diseased organs of the preoperative obese person, which serves to naturalize the health/disease distinction. It also elides the case of transition-related surgeries, among others, in which
ostensibly "healthy" body parts are surgically altered, if not made "diseased" (see
Meyerowitz 2002).

Unlike in the case of Viagra, there is no clear evidence that weight-loss surgeries have been used in radically nonnormative ways. In "On Fatness and Fluidity," Kathleen LeBesco suggests one way in which weight-loss surgeries might
be used to disrupt norms, floating the possibility that we might be able to
"sizef*ck" (based on the concept of genderf*cking) by intentionally changing
from fat to thin or thin to fat (LeBesco 2016, 52). Based on this, I can imagine a
performance artist like Orlan gaining weight, undergoing bariatric surgery (perhaps without accompanying surgery to remove "excess" skin), and then gaining
weight again, as part of a radical performance piece. However, such a performance would need to be carefully designed because, as LeBesco argues, most
people who lose and gain weight (even intentionally) will be read by society as
ambitious dieters and/or sad regainers, thus participating in, rather than challenging, existing norms (LeBesco 2016, 52).

While the above is mostly speculative, in reality, weight-loss interventions can
lead to at least some disruption of self and/or society, if not normative transgression. Cressida Heyes argues that there could be some subversive aspects to
weight loss. Heyes points out that Foucault identifies dieting practices in ancient
Greece as a "technology of the self." According to Heyes, the commercial weight-
loss company Weight Watchers actually promotes some practices that resemble
the self-care dieting practices lauded by Foucault, although Weight Watchers
ultimately exploits these discourses in the service of commercial gain and normalization. Still, Heyes argues that "real" Weight Watchers participants do not
fully accede to the disciplinary demands of the company: "In the world of meet-
ings, however, the real women I met were often aware that they could learn
from Weight Watchers without becoming the projected unified subject of its
regime" (Heyes 2006, 146). Heyes argues that feminists could potentially take
advantage of this fissure: "Central to this awareness is the possibility of uncou-
pling new capacities from docility, and of recruiting those capacities to care of
the self" (Heyes 2006, 146).

Taking this argument in a different direction, based on her own experience of using a starvation diet to transform from what she calls a "morbidly obese" black woman to a "slender" black woman, Sharrell D. Luckett develops the term "trans-weight" to "identify someone who willfully acquires a new size identity by losing or gaining a large amount of weight in a short amount of time" (Luckett 2014, 2). Luckett argues that this transformation led her into a liminal space. She writes, "The liminal space I am speaking of is one in which my mind manifests in both a fat body and slender body on a daily basis. Though I've physically crossed a border, I am trapped by psychological borders, thus my reintegration, or transformation, is incomplete . . . I constantly oscillate among these liminal spaces. I am always in between entities and never feel as though I'm one integrated self" (Luckett 2014, 5). Based on her experiences in this liminal space, Luckett developed a performance piece titled *YoungGiftedandFat* in which she performs three characters—"Fat," "Skinny," and "Sharrell." According to Luckett, the performance piece explores complicated intersections of race, sexuality, gender, and size, while simultaneously refusing easy answers and "beckoning collective resistance" (Luckett 2014).

I think it is certainly possible to argue that weight-loss medical interventions potentially undermine the association of thinness with moral rectitude. If medical/surgical interventions allow people to move into the category of thinness without "work" (note: this is not currently the case), the idea that a thin body signifies discipline and morality (and, thus, indirectly class) may lose its current grip on society. Patricia Drew argues that while diet and exercise are lauded by the media as ways to lose weight (as diet and exercise are thought to reflect self-discipline), bariatric surgery is often depicted negatively in the media as a "risky" and "extravagant procedure" that allows people an "easy escape" from fat. Therefore, according to Drew, "obesity surgery patients thus deviate from social standards in two ways: they do not have acceptable bodies and they do not transform their bodies by conventional, appropriate means" (P. Drew 2011, 1235). Suzanne Koven similarly argues that many primary-care physicians do not like to prescribe weight-loss drugs in part because they view fat people as lazy and as lacking willpower (Koven 2013).

Still, while weight loss may, in some cases, lead to a productive disruption of self and/or society, in most cases, weight loss is not a revolutionary act but a compromised and compromising strategy for surviving in an imperfect world. Based on interviews with thirty-five people in England and Scotland who had either undergone or were about to undergo weight-loss surgeries, Karen Throsby argues that weight-loss patients can be committed to neoliberal projects of normalization—her interviewees understood their weight-loss surgeries as the moment when they decided to take "decisive action," accept responsibility for their body size, and engage in work to achieve a thin self. Simultaneously, her interviewees recognized that their decision to lose weight through surgery, and not diet and exercise alone, was a stigmatized choice, and they worked hard to both manage stigma and conceal the fact of their surgeries. Throsby also points out that, similarly to transition-related care, before accessing surgery, potential weight-loss patients must demonstrate that they are committed to an understanding of obesity as a chronic health problem and are willing to spend a lifetime dieting and exercising if granted surgery. In both cases, the medical profession promotes normalization through its power as a surgical gatekeeper (Throsby 2007, 2008). In general, qualitative research with people who are undergoing or have undergone weight-loss surgeries finds that motivations for pursuing surgery are mixed but are usually related to the stigmatization of fat bodies in addition to concerns about health, and reactions to surgery are also mixed—with some experiencing the results of surgery as almost entirely positive or entirely negative, but with most experiencing the results as both positive and negative (Warholm, Øien, and Råheim 2014; P. Drew 2011; Temple Newhook, Gregory, and Twells 2015; J. Young and Burrows 2013).

A (perhaps surprising) number of fat studies/feminist scholars have written theoretically informed personal accounts of their own efforts to lose weight (Murray 2005; Longhurst 2012; Heyes 2006; see also Donaghue and Clemitshaw 2012; see also "A 'Fat Studies' Scholar No Longer Fits the Picture" 2006; see also Meleo-Erwin 2011). For example, Samantha Murray describes how she was initially joyful upon discovering the Fat Liberation movement but eventually found herself unable to feel pride in her fat body, in part because "coming out" as fat did not, for her, overcome her own tacit body knowledges, which had been indelibly shaped by the negative "knowledge" of fatness in our culture. She writes, "I came to the realization that I couldn't 'do' [Marilyn] Wann's fat politics. . . . This understanding of the self as the engineer of the body suggests that we can just change our mind about our fatness, deciding to reinscribe the meaning of our own fat. Yet, at the same time, this perception distances the fat woman even further from her own body" (Murray 2005, 275). About dieting, Murray writes, "I struggle with the guilt of compromising my theory and my politics by engaging in processes such as the diet which has me buying into the very discourses I critique, despite my awareness that it is not that easy just to 'decide' not to be affected by these dominant bodily discourses" (Murray 2005, 275). Other scholars have described similar ambivalences about engaging in weight-loss efforts. About her decision to join Weight Watchers, Cressida Heyes writes, "Suffice to say I was both interested in losing weight, embarrassed by that desire, and curious about institutionalized weight-loss programs" (Heyes 2006, 127). Robyn Longhurst describes her own pursuit of weight loss as ambivalent and paradoxical on at least three accounts:

> The first paradox is that for the last couple of years I have wrestled with critiquing discourses around women and slimness while desiring to be slim. . . .
> The second way in which losing weight has positioned me paradoxically is that I have become simultaneously a disordered and a disciplined body. . . . My own

behaviors—being acutely aware of every scrap of food or sip of drink that enters my mouth, getting on scales daily and feeling incredibly anxious about regaining weight—mark my body paradoxically as both compliant and resistant, disciplined and disordered. . . . A third way in which my shrinking body came to be positioned paradoxically was in relation to health . . . it is somewhat contradictory that when I decided to attempt to become slimmer I found myself much more focused on weight loss and what the scales said than on becoming healthy. This seemed to run counter to what I have argued publicly as a feminist academic. (Longhurst 2012, 882)

These theoretically informed testimonies suggest that while many people may, indeed, learn to love, embrace, and celebrate their fatness, even some fat-positive feminists attempt weight loss. These attempts may be motivated by "health" reasons, by an inability to overcome a lifetime of negative messages about fat combined with the ongoing stigmatization of fat bodies, and/or by an inability to reject the appeal of developing a body that is not the object of hate.

In her article titled "'A Beautiful Show of Strength': Weight Loss and the Fat Activist Self," Zoë C. Meleo-Erwin analyses two online accounts of weight loss by fat activists—Hanne Blank's blog about her efforts to lose weight titled "The Fickle Finger of Fat: A Reduced-Fat Blog for the Large of Brain" and a guest post on the fat activist blog "Shapely Prose" by "Heidi" about her decision to have weight-loss surgery. According to Meleo-Erwin, Blank and Heidi both affirmed their critique of fat phobia while also using discourses of agency and autonomy to defend their right to pursue fat reduction/weight-loss surgery in order to improve their own well-being. Meleo-Erwin also analyzes the responses to Blank and Heidi's posts, noting that while there was criticism, particularly of Heidi, both activists also received a lot of support from fat activist communities. I find much to commend in both Blank and Heidi's approaches and am gladdened by the support they received from fat-positive communities. However, Meleo-Erwin notes a trend in the response to Blank and Heidi that I find problematic:

As with Blank's commenters, many of those who responded to Heidi's post began to frame their support of her decision by differentiating between legitimate, informed and empowered weight loss decisions and those which are made from a place of internalized fat-phobia . . . by making recourse to discussions of agency and autonomy, Blank, Heidi and their responders produce the fat activist as someone who, while still being critical of weight loss industries, can make the choice to pursue weight loss so long as this choice is grounded in both a larger ethic of fat positivity and in a true state of bodily impairment. (Meleo-Erwin 2011, 200)

As should hopefully be clear by now, this is a move I wish to reject—there is not some line that can be drawn between empowered weight-loss decisions and those made from a place of internalized fat phobia (we are all socialized in a fat-phobic society and none of us are immune from the effects), and there is no clear line between a true state of bodily impairment and a disability that results from social structures. Thus, while I too affirm here the right of people to choose to pursue weight-loss interventions in order to live a more fulfilling life and certainly agree that there could be more or less problematic cases of weight loss, I do not believe it is possible to neatly separate out "pure" motives from "impure" ones.

While some may be troubled by the implicit/explicit comparison made by Luckett between weight-loss interventions and transition-related medical interventions for trans people, I believe the comparison is worth exploring, if only to clarify similarities and differences between the two cases. The cases seem different. Weight loss (when successful) only ever moves people from a stigmatized category (fat) to a privileged category (thin), thus validating, at a social level, the desirability of thinness. Transition-related care, however, can move people from a stigmatized category or categories (gender nonconforming and/or female) to a privileged category or categories (gender conforming and/or male) but can also move people from a privileged category or categories (gender conforming and/or male) to a marginalized category or categories (gender nonconforming and/or female). Thus, transition-related interventions seem to have a more complicated relationship to regimes of normalization than weight-loss interventions. However, as I argued in a previous chapter, ultimately we want to affirm the right of trans people to access transition-related interventions that promote self-flourishing, even when these interventions sometimes align with regimes of normalization, and I believe that a similar argument can be made in the case of weight-loss interventions.

Evaluating medical weight-loss interventions through the lens of a perspective that combines the best of feminist/fat-positive and critical public health approaches allows us to see that fat people can be caught in a double bind—our social, political, and built environments produce fatness and differentially distribute it according to social categories of power and privilege while simultaneously discriminating against and stigmatizing fat people. Our priority as feminists should be to work to end discrimination and stigma against fat people while altering the unjust aspects of our world that differentially distribute fatness. At the same time, we can understand that while some/many fat people may be able to embrace their fatness in this world, others may find themselves unable to overcome negative tacit body knowledges inculcated by society and/or may be unable to survive the everyday discrimination directed at fat people. In these latter cases, weight loss may be a necessary survival strategy. In addition, to the extent that acute thinness and acute heaviness in some cases do seem to have significant "health-related" consequences, it may be the case that some acutely heavy people do experience significant health benefits from weight loss.[22] Given the enormous difficulty of losing weight through diet and exercise options, weight-loss interventions such as weight-loss pharmaceuticals and bariatric surgeries may actually be the most effective interventions in terms of producing long-term weight loss. In addition, weight-loss pharmaceuticals and bariatric surgeries are, in some ways, less aligned than diet and exercise with Puritan and neoliberal calls for personal responsibility and hard (self) work.[23]

Conclusion

In this chapter, I have examined feminist and fat-positive critiques of our cultural obsession with slenderness and of fat phobia. I have also examined critical public health approaches to weight, which argue that fat is produced by the physical, political, economic, and social architecture of our society and is differentially distributed along lines of gender, race, class, and ability, among others. I have argued that combining the two approaches leads to a more complete understanding of the social construction of weight and encourages us, as feminists, to focus on challenging stigma and discrimination against fat people while also transforming our society to promote access to more-nutritious food and opportunities for physical activity and to reduce stress, environmental toxins, and other causes of weight gain.

I have also argued that combining these two approaches can lead us to rethink our evaluation of medical and surgical approaches to weight loss. These procedures are certainly undergirded by and promote fat phobia. At the same time, they may improve health for people who are acutely heavy, and they may be an understandable option for others who find their ability to flourish in this society severely limited due to their weight. Thus, even though I have even more reservations about weight-loss medications and surgeries than about the transition-related interventions discussed in Chapter 3 and the sexuopharmaceuticals discussed in Chapter 4, ultimately I come down on a similar position— focus on transforming larger structures of oppression, put systems in place to ameliorate some of the negative social and political effects of normalizing medical interventions, and also allow individuals to access normalizing medical interventions if they decide, in consultation with their communities, that these interventions are the best available route to their survival and/or flourishing.

CHAPTER 6

Conclusion

MEDICINE WITHOUT EUGENICS?

In this book, I have attempted to demonstrate that it is often difficult to take a "for" or "against" position against specific medical interventions. The three interventions I have analyzed—transition-related interventions, sexuopharmaceuticals, and weight-loss interventions—are different in many ways. In some ways, transition-related interventions are always norm-transgressing, in that they enable trans individuals to move away from the gender categories they were assigned at birth. Sexuopharmaceuticals are intended to be used and are likely used in the majority of cases in norm-congruent ways. Yet, they do seem to be used in a significant minority of cases in norm-transgressing ways. In contrast, medical weight-loss interventions are used almost exclusively in norm-confirming ways, although the fact that they seem to offer a "quick fix" challenges certain puritanical norms.

In addition, while gender transitioning has attained legitimacy in some circles, it remains stigmatized by a majority of Americans (A. Brown 2017). While Viagra and erectile dysfunction (ED) remain the subject of much joking, the use of male ED drugs has been consistently destigmatized over the past two decades (Vares and Braun 2006; J. R. Fishman 2009). By contrast, while interventions to lose weight in general are commonly practiced and highly praised, medical weight-loss interventions are stigmatized (P. Drew 2011; Koven 2013).

Transition-related medical interventions are also sought by a relatively small percentage of the population (Sifferlin 2017). In contrast, male sexuopharmaceuticals are consumed by millions of users and produce billions of dollars in profits (Mukherjee 2018). While some expected female sexuopharmaceuticals to be similarly popular and profitable, so far that has not proved to be the case (Cohen 2018). Medical weight-loss interventions fall in between the two extremes, but they are part of a larger, and hugely profitable, weight-loss industry (M. Martin et al. 2010).

Finally, it is clear that transition-related care can save lives, as studies have shown that trans people who have undergone gender-reassignment interventions report fewer suicide attempts after medically transitioning (Murad et al. 2010). In contrast, while it is certainly true that sexual dissatisfaction can be extremely distressing, it is unlikely that sexuopharmaceuticals are "life-saving" in the way that transition-related care can be. Medical weight-loss interventions may be more similar to transition-related interventions in this sense—these interventions can reduce death from a variety of conditions such as diabetes and heart attack, and they may also reduce suicide rates (Chang et al. 2014).

Yet, despite these significant differences, these three types of medical interventions share some things in common. In each case, they can be used—and often are used—to bring bodies/minds into conformity with social norms—be those related to binary gender, heterosexuality, or thinness. In each case, the interventions have the potential to be used in norm-transgressing ways, even if weight-loss interventions are not currently used this way. In addition, in all three cases, the interventions do have the potential to reduce some individual suffering and make some lives more livable.

In general, like other technologies, medical interventions are developed and implemented within a society structured by inequalities: of race, gender, sexuality, ability, nationality, and more. Not surprisingly, therefore, medical interventions are often intended by their developers and used by those who have access to them to (attempt) to produce bodies/minds that more closely resemble what Rosemarie Garland-Thomson calls "the normate" (Garland-Thomson 1997). At the same time, extremely marginalized individuals are often unable to access the medical interventions that are necessary to maintain life.

Still, medical interventions are also usually employed by a minority of users to achieve nonnormative ends, and even when they are employed to achieve normative ends, medical interventions can make life more livable and can sometimes allow people to live more fulfilling lives in a deeply unjust society. I have argued that it is this contradictory reality that has led to a repeated cycling within feminist, antiracist, queer, and disability-affirming activism and scholarship between denunciations and affirmations of medical interventions, particularly those that most obviously involve issues of class, race, gender, sexuality, ability, and other social categories related to privilege and oppression. It has been my argument that because this cycling is the result of a contradictory reality, a "for" or "against" position will not eventually be discovered through further refining our theoretical tools or through developing greater analytical clarity.

As a result, I have suggested that one possible response that would move us away from this cyclical pattern is to make a threefold move: first, to allow individuals, in consultation with their communities and with certain safeguards in place, to decide for themselves whether to use a particular intervention; to create a feminist democratic system for making decisions about healthcare and determining which interventions should be covered by insurance; and, third, to focus our political energies on addressing the broader sociopolitical structures that currently ensure that medical interventions are used largely in the service of normalization and working to ensure that all people, regardless of race, gender, sexuality, nation, class, or ability, have access to the basic resources required to flourish.

In this conclusion, I discuss in a more systematic and generalized way a few issues that have emerged in each of the previous chapters: I first make a general argument for replacing and supplementing the language of "medical necessity" and "pathology" with the language of fulfillment, livability, and flourishing. Using the language of fulfillment, livability, and flourishing, I then offer a more general discussion of the threefold move mentioned above (individual decision making, feminist democratic processes for determining public funding, and social/structural activism). Finally, I grapple with the issue of whether medical interventions are necessarily eugenicist.

The Language of Pathology and Medical Necessity

As discussed in Chapter 2, there is still significant debate among scholars over how to define illness and where to draw the line between sickness and health. As noted in that chapter, some scholars have argued that we should develop a "naturalistic" account of disease, such that, for example, disease is defined as deviation from "species-typical functioning" (Boorse 1975). However, as a number of critics have pointed out, "species-typical functioning" cannot be established objectively, and even if it could be, equating what is "natural" with what is "healthy" relies on a problematic value judgment (Kingma 2007, 2014). Others have argued for a "normative" account of disease, arguing that disease is a socially constructed category and that we must define it explicitly based on our values (e.g., Sparrow 2013b). However, as my discussion of Sparrow's work suggests, in addition to other problems, normative accounts tend to pathologize at least some who do not wish to be pathologized and leave "unpathologized" some who might want to benefit from medical intervention (Gupta and Freeman 2013).

The situation is complicated by the fact that in the United States, at least, the words "pathology," "disease," and "disorder" carry and confer stigma. More than two decades ago, Susan Wendell identified a primary cause of this stigma—our society's idolization of the perfect body and our belief in the endless perfectibility of the body, as well as our resulting fear and refusal of bodily impairment, vulnerability, and death (Wendell 1989). Wendell writes,

> Suffering caused by the body, and the inability to control the body, are despised, pitied, and, above all, feared. This fear, experienced individually, is also deeply embedded in our culture. . . . The disabled are not only de-valued for their

de-valued bodies, they are constant reminders to the able-bodied of the negative body—of what the able-bodied are trying to avoid, forget and ignore.
For example, if someone tells me she is in pain, she reminds me of the existence of pain, the imperfection and fragility of the body, the possibility of my
own pain, the inevitability of it. . . . Gradually, I make her 'other' because I
don't want to confront my real body, which I fear and cannot accept. (Wendell
1989, 112–113)

Disability and illness also threaten one's economic independence and productivity, which again are deeply held American values and, in the absence of a
comprehensive social safety net, are often necessary for simple survival. For
these reasons, in American history, disability has often been equated with or
even defined as the inability to support oneself economically (Schweik 2009;
Nielsen 2012).

The stigma associated with disease, along with the process of medicalizing
bodily and mental states that fall outside the "norm" but that do not necessarily
require medical intervention, has led to a complicated political situation. On one
hand, individuals, activists, and scholars from pathologized groups who do not
want to alter their bodies or minds through medical interventions very understandably argue that they are not, in fact, disordered and lobby to eliminate diagnoses that suggest that their way of being-in-the-world is, in some way, necessarily imperfect. In recent history, there have been many examples of people from
pathologized groups rejecting the label of pathology, disorder, and/or disability—
including "homosexuals" who fought for the removal of homosexuality from
the *Diagnostic and Statistical Manual of Mental Disorders* (*DSM*) (Bayer 1987),
those members of the Deaf community who will not use the label of "disability"
to describe deafness (L. J. Davis 1995), some trans activists who seek to eliminate the diagnosis of gender dysphoria from the *DSM* (see Chapter 3), some asexual activists who argue that asexuality is not a disorder (see Chapter 4), and
some fat-pride activists who argue that fatness should not be considered a disease
(see Chapter 5), among others. This argument is, in part, entirely appropriate—
if medical intervention is not needed or desired, why should members of a
socially marginalized group receive a medical label?

On the other hand, the quest for depathologization can have (often unin-
tended) negative consequences. For one thing, it can be an essentializing argument—to assert that one knows oneself to be "not sick," "not disordered," or "not
disabled," suggests that one can know what it means to be "sick," "disordered,"
or "disabled"—in other words, that these social categories have ascertainable
borders. In addition, it suggests that the conditions "left behind" in the realm of
pathologization are "inherently disordered" when, in fact, disability studies
scholarship suggests that all "pathological" conditions are, to some extent, produced by the interaction between body/mind and environment.

At the same time, the quest for depathologization is often also motivated by a desire to escape the stigma associated with pathology, which, although understandable, does not challenge the stigma itself, leaving it in place for those individuals and groups who remain within pathologized categories. Even if the quest for depathologization is not about escaping stigma, the very intensity with which many activists pursue depathologization can send the message that the problem is not just that a categorization mistake has been made but that there is something undesirable about the category into which one has been placed.

In addition, this move can lead to the marginalization of individuals who belong to the group that some are seeking to depathologize and who also need or desire medical labels or interventions for other aspects of their mind/body—in other words, for example, a person who identifies as asexual and who has an autoimmune condition may feel uncomfortable with the assertion that "asexual people are not sick" (E. Kim 2010, 2011; Gupta 2014). In addition, it can become difficult when some members of a community do not need or desire medical interventions (and seek depathologization) while other members do need or desire medical interventions—clearly this is the case for trans communities (explored in Chapter 3) but also for a number of other pathologized categories—such as autism, where some people with autism seek depathologization and demedicalization in favor of a "neurodiversity" model, whereas others seek specific kinds of medical interventions to address specific "symptoms" (this example is complicated, of course, by the fact that it is often caregivers who seek medical interventions for children with autism) (S. M. Robertson 2009; Runswick-Cole 2014; Grandin n.d.). In these cases, it can prove difficult to depathologize parts of the community while leaving medical labels and interventions in place for other members of the community.

Scholars and activists have productively challenged the naturalization and stigmatization of disease categories from multiple directions. A number of scholars and activists have argued that everyone is only "temporarily abled" or always already "becoming disabled"—if we live long enough, we will inevitably develop some form of physical or mental disability (Garland-Thomson 2012). Along these lines, feminist legal scholar Martha Fineman has argued that we should focus on universal dependency and vulnerability when designing our society in order to promote social justice (Albertson Fineman 2008). Scholars and activists have also reclaimed disease and illness labels as markers of pride—many people in the disability rights movement self-identify with labels such as "crippled," "mad," "autie," and, indeed, "disabled" (for a discussion, see Clare, Spade, and Morales 2015). In addition to arguing that there is nothing inherently worse about nonnormative forms of embodiment, many activists and scholars have argued that living in the world as a person with an illness or disability can lead to a unique and valuable perspective, or disability standpoint (Wendell 2013; Garland-Thomson 2012; Mairs 1997; Kleege 1999). In "The Case for Conserving

Disability," Garland-Thomson argues that disability is a narrative resource, an epistemological resource, and an ethical resource (Garland-Thomson 2012), a point that I will return to later in this chapter.

For all of these reasons, in this work, I have advocated for abandoning the framework of health and illness altogether in favor of the language of fulfillment, livability, and flourishing. By fulfillment, I mean something along the lines of the ability to live in a way that brings one satisfaction, which means that what it means to live a fulfilling life will look different for different people.[1] In this more phenomenological model, certain aspects of our minds or bodies (in interaction with the world) may be hindering our ability to flourish and certain medical interventions might improve our ability to flourish. We might still need and want to come up with names and descriptions of particular states so we can evaluate the extent to which particular medical interventions might be effective at altering that specific state in a specific way.

To the extent that two people might share similar forms of bodies or minds (states), it is entirely possible that the flourishing of one might be promoted by a medical intervention while the flourishing of the other might be harmed by the same medical intervention. This model does not presume the cause of a particular form of embodiment or mindfulness (apart from the assumption that minds/bodies are produced through the iterative interaction of biology and society), and it does not presume that medical interventions are the best or only way to improve our ability to live a fulfilling life—in some cases, altering society may be the better option or both medical and societal interventions might be pursued simultaneously.

I am not suggesting that this is a perfect model for thinking and talking about medical interventions or that this should become the one single model, but it is one alternative way of conceptualizing medical interventions that can help to avoid some of the political problems discussed above. In particular, in this model, no particular type of mind/body is inherently disordered or healthy, and any particular type of mind/body could be problematic or not, depending on the person and the context. In addition, this model does not automatically lump entire groups of people with similar types of minds/bodies together in a group deemed either healthy or pathological but rather acknowledges that some people may find a particular form of mind/body to be in need of alteration while others may find a similar form of mind/body configuration to be perfectly congruent with flourishing. To give just one overly simplified concrete illustration, under this model, for example, we might talk about deafness and "hearingness" as two forms of mind/body existence, both of which may be problematic for some (who might wish to pursue medical interventions to increase or decrease auditory capacities) but not for others. Obviously, of course, the current configuration of our society means that deafness is much more likely to be experienced as problematic than hearingness.

Threefold Move

Throughout this book, I have advocated for a threefold move on the part of feminist activists and scholars: allowing for individual decision making, creating feminist democratic processes for making decisions about healthcare, and engaging in activism to transform our society as a whole. Here I discuss each of these moves using the language of flourishing, livability, and fulfillment.

Individual Decision Making

First, I have argued that whether a particular medical intervention is important for a person's flourishing will depend on the individual person and the context of her life. For this reason, I have argued that we should allow individuals, in consultation with their communities, to decide for themselves whether to use a particular intervention, even if they intend to use the intervention in the service of normalization.

As feminist ethicists have long pointed out, humans are not isolated individuals. Human identity is relational, and we are bound to others (humans and nonhumans) in complicated webs. While I do not believe there is any practical way to require individuals to consider their relational others when they make decisions about medical interventions, I believe we could implement standards of care such that individuals are encouraged to consult, or at least consider, their communities before making medical decisions.

At the same time, because it is clear that individuals, even in consultation with their communities, will tend to make medical decisions that reinforce, rather than challenge, unjust social norms, I believe that we should implement some guidelines that may at least temper these outcomes. For example, in an earlier work, when discussing the ethics of using medical or pharmacological interventions to change sexual desires or attachments, I argued that the availability of these interventions could lead to a reduction in sexual diversity. At the same time, I offered a list of suggestions that could potentially limit the extent to which these interventions would be used to reduce sexual diversity, such as requiring medical professionals who are prescribing these interventions to provide their patients with information about sexual diversity and referrals to appropriate sexual communities (i.e., BDSM communities) (Gupta 2012). I think it is possible that similar guidelines could be developed for other medical interventions. To give just one more hypothetical example, we might require doctors performing bariatric surgery to provide patients with referrals to fat-positive online communities and information about the Health at Every Size movement before performing surgery. It is my hope that these kinds of guidelines could mitigate some of the ill effects of allowing individuals to make choices within a society structured by inequality. However, it is unlikely that these kinds of restrictions will make a major difference—I would still expect most people to use medical interventions to bring their minds/bodies into closer alignment with norms, which will lead to the reduction of mind/body diversity and, in some cases, the elimination of certain ways of being-in-the-world.

Feminist Democratic Decision Making about the
Health Care System and Public Funding

Feminist scholars have long argued that feminist principles support the need for a single-payer healthcare system (H. L. Nelson and Nelson 2013; Norsigian 1993). However, as feminist scholars have also argued, transitioning to a single-payer system will not eliminate the need to make decisions about what kinds of medical interventions will be developed and which medical interventions will be funded and which will not, and it is unlikely that society will be able to develop and fund all of the medical interventions that could promote an individual's flourishing. As Nelson writes, "Even the best arguments supporting the claim that there is a right to healthcare are not able to determine just how much and what kind of healthcare people are entitled to by virtue of that right, as distribution simply on the basis of need is either impossible (since the need is in principle unlimited) or is itself unjust (since the attempt to provide care on the basis of need would undermine the provision of other goods to which claims of right can be made)" (J. L. Nelson 1996, 53).

So, how should decisions about healthcare funding be made, and how would these decisions be conceptualized if the model of disease/illness is replaced with the language of flourishing/fulfillment? I argue that feminist democratic processes will need to be put in place to determine what kinds of interventions to develop and which interventions should be funded. There is a significant body of scholarship on feminist democratic theory, and it is beyond the scope of this book to engage with all of the debates in this field. However, what seems to be common to this work is the idea that feminist democratic systems will involve deliberation and the solicitation of the agreement of others, without the appeal to metaphysical truths or foundations. According to this scholarship, feminist democratic systems will enable fields of interaction where multiple axes of difference, identity, and subordination intersect, but processes must be put in place in order to ensure that the voices of marginalized individuals and groups can be heard. Finally, much of feminist democratic theory recognizes that democratic contestation is a continual process that will constantly remake subjectivities, identities, and political projects (see McAfee and Snyder 2007; I. M. Young 2002; Zerilli 2005).

In terms of determining whether a particular medical intervention will be funded, in the current disease/illness model, in the United States, in order to access a publicly or privately covered medical intervention, a person must conform to one of a finite list of bodily or mental states (deemed pathological or disordered), and this conformation must be verified by a medical professional (i.e., it must be authoritatively diagnosed). In other words, as an example, a person must have a particular body mass index (BMI), confirmed by a medical professional, in order to obtain medical insurance coverage of bariatric surgery. In general, health insurance (whether public or private) is supposed to cover those procedures deemed "medically necessary" by medical professionals. Of course, what is deemed "medically necessary" changes over time, not just with the development of new understandings of the mind/body and new medical interventions but also with changing social norms. For example, as mentioned in Chapter 3, in 2014, Medicare (government-run health insurance for older Americans) began to cover transition-related care when "medically necessary" ("Medicare" n.d.). Of course, even when medical interventions are deemed "medically necessary," they may still be inaccessible for people without any form of health insurance or with low-cost health insurance and even for people with comprehensive health insurance who cannot afford copays or deductibles. For example, as mentioned in a footnote to Chapter 5, research has demonstrated that among those who are considered "medically eligible" for bariatric surgery, minority individuals and low-income individuals are less likely to undergo bariatric surgery (M. Martin et al. 2010; Wallace et al. 2010).

If we replace the disease/illness model with the model of what is needed to live a fulfilling life, how would our society decide which medical interventions should be covered? Overall levels of healthcare funding would be decided democratically. In this model, individual decisions about funding would not be determined based on whether one conforms to one of a finite list of states but based on whether one is hindered in one's flourishing and whether a particular medical intervention would likely increase one's ability to flourish. Medical insurance (whether public or private) would, in theory, cover those procedures deemed sufficiently important for flourishing for a particular individual. Who would decide if a procedure is sufficiently important for the flourishing of a particular individual and on what basis? I imagine that, for purposes of convenient administration, through feminist democratic decision making, we might come up with a list of mind/body states for which specific corresponding medical interventions will always be funded if desired (e.g., broken bones and casts, respectively). However, much of the time, decisions could be made, in each individual case, by an interdisciplinary team, composed of doctors, patient advocates, public policy experts, critical theorists, and members of the public, based on whether a particular state of embodiment or mindfulness is significantly inhibiting self-defined flourishing *for that specific person* and whether a particular medical intervention is likely to increase that person's ability to flourish. At the same time, decision makers would need to take into account the likely effect of the medical intervention on the patient's community, or those she is in relationship with, and on society at large.

While this model may seem unfamiliar to many Americans, it exists in some form in other parts of the world. For example, in the United Kingdom, the

National Health Service (NHS) is not allowed to impose a "blanket ban" on specific procedures, but local commissioners are allowed to produce lists of "low-value" procedures that will not regularly be funded. However, individuals can apply to "individual funding request" (IFR) panels for "one-off" approval of "low-value" procedures (Russell, Swinglehurst, and Greenhalgh 2014). A study by Russel et al. analyzing how these panels respond to requests for breast surgery indicates that these panels tend to attempt to "objectively" adjudicate whether the procedure would be "cosmetic" or "medically necessary" for the individual, but in fact, their deliberations reveal that "health care rationing policy and practices, as interpretive acts, inevitably involve judgements of moral worth and deservingness, and can never be simply evidence-based endeavours" (Russell, Swinglehurst, and Greenhalgh 2014, 12). Under the model I am proposing, it would become the norm, rather than the exception, for decisions about healthcare funding to be made by panels. In addition, rather than attempting to arrive at some type of value-neutral decision, the panels would recognize and embrace the fact that the cases appearing before them are, in Russell et al.'s words, "complex instances of human suffering, involving moral engagement and emotionally and clinically challenging judgements" (Russell, Swinglehurst, and Greenhalgh 2014, 11).

Obviously, this system would not be perfect. In a society structured by inequality, allowing the public to decide overall levels of funding for medical services and interdisciplinary teams to make decisions about whether individual interventions will be covered will likely place marginalized individuals at risk, even with robust processes in place. There would certainly need to be a robust appeals process in place, such that people who are initially denied coverage for desired interventions could have their case reevaluated by others. Still, while this proposal is hardly perfect, I do think this model offers some potential benefits over the current way that we conceptualize public funding for healthcare.

Activism to Transform Our Society as a Whole

As should be clear by now, allowing individuals to make decisions about medical interventions, even with the caveats mentioned above, will likely lead to the perpetuation of social inequality and the reduction of mind/body diversity. Thus, as I have argued throughout this book, feminist activists and scholars must focus our attention on altering the broader structures of our society in order to create a world that promotes flourishing for all.

In each of the chapters, I offered some broader goals for feminist activists and scholars. In the chapter on transition-related care, one of my suggestions was that we should focus our efforts on changing laws so that legal rights and social services for trans people are no longer contingent on medical/surgical transitioning. In the chapter on sexuopharmaceuticals, one of my suggestions was that we should focus our efforts on providing comprehensive sexual education to all children. In the chapter on weight-loss interventions, one of my suggestions was that we should work to end discrimination against fat people, for example, by making it illegal for employers to discriminate on the basis of weight. A second suggestion was to focus our efforts on building public recreational facilities in order to give all people, regardless of ability, the opportunity to engage in physical activity if they want to. These are just a few of examples of the broader structural changes that, if enacted, will contribute both to individual flourishing and to the creation of a society in which mind/body diversity is accommodated and valued.

THE MEDICAL MODEL AND EUGENIC LOGICS

Before concluding, I wish to address the relationship between the argument I have made in this book and the critique of eugenics that has been developing within the field of disability studies. In "The Case for Conserving Disability," Rosemarie Garland-Thomson identifies the ubiquity and persistence of what she calls "eugenic logic" in modern Western thought and practice. She defines eugenic logic as follows:

> Eugenic logic tells us that our world would be a better place if disability could be eliminated. Enacted worldwide in policies and practices that range from segregation to extermination, the aim of eugenics is to eliminate disability and, by extension, disabled people from the world. Eugenic logic is a utopian effort to improve the social order, a practical health program, or a social justice initiative that is simply common sense to most people and is supported by the logic of modernity itself. . . . Why—eugenic logic asks—should the world we make and occupy together include disability at all? (Garland-Thomson 2012, 339–340)

Garland-Thomson argues that because disability is inevitable and because disability provides our society with at least three types of resources—narrative, epistemic, and ethical—we should think about disability not as something to be eliminated but as something—like ecological diversity—to be valued and preserved (Garland-Thomson 2012).

As Garland-Thomson suggests in the definition above, eugenic logic is not limited to conservative political projects and, in fact, is in some ways more present within progressive and social justice–oriented projects, as these projects aim to "make the world a better place," and it is "common sense" to most people that the world would be a better place if it contained less physical pain, less illness, less disability, and less (premature?) death. After all, as a society, we are biased against pain, suffering, and illness; we tend to underestimate the quality of life of people with disabilities; and we tend to assume that a person born with a disability or illness will not be able to live as fulfilling a life as a person born with a more "normative" form of mind/body (Garland-Thomson 2017). Alison Kafer identifies eugenic logic at work in some feminist projects; using Marge Piercy's speculative novel *Woman on the Edge of Time* (1976) as a case study, she argues that Piercy imagines a utopian world in which many kinds of diversity—including racial and sexual diversity—are accepted, but disability is almost completely absent. According to Kafer, Piercy's utopia demonstrates that even for many feminists, the better world that we imagine is a world without disability (Kafer 2013).

Certainly, allowing access to the kinds of medical interventions discussed in this book in the world as it is would likely decrease the presence of certain kinds of disability. Thus, as I have argued above, we, as a society, should implement specific safeguards in order to conserve as much bodily and mental diversity as possible as we work to change the broader structures that compel normalization.

At the same time, the many structural changes I have advocated for in this book—from decreasing stigma against people with disabilities to increasing acceptance for gender diversity—would help to conserve and may even grow and multiply some types of bodily and mental diversity. In theory, challenging the forces that compel normalization would not only enable people to refuse certain medical interventions but also allow people to use medical interventions in more creative and divergent ways—to remove "healthy" limbs and to add "extra" limbs, to develop "gendered" forms of embodiment not yet conceived of, to reduce certain sensory inputs and to acquire new ways of obtaining sensory input, to select both for and against "disability" using assistive reproductive technologies, and so forth—things that happen now, but only on a very small scale.

And yet, many feminist, antiracist, and queer political projects aimed at altering the broader structures of our society would also potentially reduce the presence of disability in the world. To the extent that disability is produced by war, imperialism, colonialism, poverty, environmental pollution, antiblack police brutality, unrealistic beauty standards that differentially impact women, violence against LGBTQ+ people, and more forms of discriminatory violence, then feminist, antiracist, and queer political projects that seek to eliminate these forms of oppression will possibly have eugenic effects, even if they are not motivated primarily by the desire to eliminate disability from the world. Certainly, the kinds of public health interventions discussed in Chapter 5—such as increasing access to "more nutritious" food and opportunities for physical recreation while reducing the amount of carcinogens in our food and water—might lead to a decrease in certain forms of physical disability. How do we reconcile this with Garland-Thomson's call for conserving disability?

One valid way of reconciling these competing claims would be to argue that we should only pursue social justice projects that are justified by goals other than reducing pain, illness, disability, and death—in other words, we oppose antiblack police violence because it is unjust, not because it produces pain, illness, and death. Another potential option is to argue that these processes that produce disability, such as war, racism, environmental destruction, and so on, simultaneously produce trauma, and it is really the trauma, and not necessarily the disability itself, that we are attempting to eliminate. A third appealing response (and one consonant with this book's embrace of contradictions) would be to argue that we must simply acknowledge that it is a contradiction to simultaneously value existing disabled lives while also attempting to end some processes that bring those lives into existence, but that this contradiction is one that we must live with. In addition to accepting these responses, I also take a slightly different tack. While Garland-Thomson identifies the drive to eliminate suffering entirely as a distinctly modernist impulse, I do not believe we should therefore take the exact opposite position of accepting all pain, illness, suffering, and death. Rather, we must once again adopt a more contingent position that affords us less certainty—some types of pain and illness might be worth conserving for some or all, and some might be worth reducing or eliminating for some or all.

In addition, while I agree completely with the intent behind Garland-Thomson's call to preserve disability, I would want to suggest that while we should absolutely be focused on preserving mind/body diversity and might want to work to preserve particular disability cultures (e.g., Deaf cultures that have developed their own languages, literatures, and, indeed, knowledge systems), we also should be hesitant to become too entrenched in our defense of any one particular form of mind/body existence. To put this more plainly, there are certain forms of minds/bodies that are no longer in existence—for example, smallpox has been virtually eliminated through vaccination, leading to the elimination of people with smallpox scars—while other forms of mind/body are of recent origin—for example, people living with artificial hearts—and it seems to me that, as the world changes, there will inevitably be change in terms of what forms of embodiment/mindfulness exist. Because I think this kind of change is inevitable, I think we must be able to acknowledge and mourn lost forms of mind/body existence while also remaining open to as yet unknown future forms of mind/body existence.

Based on this reasoning, I argue that we do need to challenge eugenic logic in progressive projects while working to create a world that embraces mind/body diversity, including what is currently thought of as "disability." However, I do not think this commits us to conserving every form of mind/body currently in existence. Indeed, the project of conserving biodiversity, from which Garland-Thomson explicitly draws her language, can be focused on preserving either individual species or the ecosystem *processes* that allow for biological and species diversity, or both. In addition, most environmentalists argue that conserving biodiversity is one goal that must be balanced with and/or against others, from providing social and economic opportunities for marginalized people to preserving "ecosystem services" (a conservation goal different from the goal of conserving biodiversity) (Faith 2016; McShane et al. 2011). Thus, I argue that we should challenge eugenic logic by creating and preserving the *processes* that enable the flourishing of mind/body diversity of various kinds (including gender, sexual, racial, ethnic, and ability/disability) while also recognizing that the preservation of mind/body diversity is one among many goals of social justice activism. Processes that enable the flourishing of mind/body diversity include many of the proposals mentioned already, such as sexual education systems that promote sexual diversity, legal processes that prohibit employment discrimination on the basis of any personal characteristic that is not related to inherent job requirements, and the establishment of diverse decision-making bodies in the healthcare field.

Disability studies scholars rightly criticize those who suggest that disabled lives are "not worth living."[2] But, we must also recognize that there is no way to avoid deciding who should and should not inhabit the world or which lives are worth living and which are not worth living. We constantly make decisions— as individuals and as a society—that affect both the quality of life of people currently living and the shape (literally and figuratively) of people to come—from decisions as small as what to eat for breakfast to as large as whether to fund research into a cure for HIV/AIDS or a vaccine for HIV/AIDS, or both. Not acknowledging that we constantly make decisions about which lives are worth living is a decision in itself. Currently, these decisions are shaped by ableism, sexism, heterosexism, racism, imperialism, colonialism, and other forms of injustice. The goal is not, and cannot be, to create a society in which these decisions do not have to be made but to create a society in which these decisions can be made democratically and free from engrained systems of social inequality.

POTENTIAL FOR COALITION BUILDING

Feminists of color have argued that coalition politics are a dangerous but necessary business (Fowlkes 1997; Yuval-Davis 1993). Drawing from women of color theorists, particularly Chela Sandoval, Donna Haraway argues that coalition politics cannot be formed on the basis of "natural identification" but only "on the basis of conscious coalition, of affinity, of political kinship" (Haraway 1991b, 156). According to Haraway, this work of coalition building benefits from an embrace of irony. Haraway writes, "Irony is about contradictions that do not resolve into larger wholes, even dialectically, about the tension of holding incompatible things together because both or all are necessary and true" (Haraway 1991b, 149).

In attempting to hold together unresolvable contradictions, it is my hope that the analysis and strategies offered in this project will facilitate coalition building across difference. In this book, I have identified a number of sites where coalitions are being built or could/should be built: between reproductive rights

activists and disability activists; between trans activists and reproductive justice activists, between asexual activists and disability activists, and between fat-
positive feminists, public health officials, labor organizers, animal rights activ-
ists, and environmental justice activists, among others. I have also tried to engage
in the kind of interdisciplinary critique that can enable coalition formation
between scholars across disciplines. In general, in refusing to settle on a simple
for or against position, it is my hope that the approach offered in this book will
provide space for people with conflicting priorities and desires to be able to both
pursue their own agenda and to find common cause in working to dismantle
the overarching systems of oppression that hinder everyone's ability to flourish.

MEDICINE IS NOT SPECIAL

I want to conclude by suggesting that medical interventions are not inherently
different from a variety of individual survival or advancement strategies that aim
to increase the quality of one's own life (or the life or lives of one's immediate
family and friends) in a deeply unjust society—including private education,
migration, and employment, among others. In an unjust society, pursuit of individual well-being often means conforming to, reinforcing, and perhaps propa-
gating inequalities based on race, gender, sexuality, ability, and so on. For those
with more privilege, individual strategies can sometimes lead to significant
advancement. For those with less privilege, individual strategies may be the only
way to survive. And many individuals will be too disenfranchised or will lack
the resources to pursue individual strategies at all. At the same time, individual
strategies can be and are used in a minority of cases in antinormative, resistant,
or even transformative ways.

My argument in this book, then, essentially boils down to this—be critical
of individual survival and advancement strategies but do not eliminate them as
options. At the same time, implement safeguards in order to mitigate the worst
systemic effects of individual efforts to pursue survival and flourishing in an
unjust society. Survival is a necessary and important goal. Reflecting on her life
in the months following her breast surgery after receiving a diagnosis of breast
cancer, Audre Lorde writes, "We [Black women] have had to learn this first and
most vital lesson—that we were never meant to survive. Not as human beings"
(Lorde 1984, 42). In A Burst of Light, Lorde writes, "Caring for myself is not self-
indulgence, it is self-preservation, and that is an act of political warfare" (Lorde
2017, 130).

And yet, individual survival, and even individual flourishing, can never be
our only goal. We, as feminist scholars and activists, must dedicate ourselves to
changing the broader unjust structures of society. For Lorde, survival itself
always entails political action—in order for the individual to survive, she must
pursue collective action to transform society. In "The Master's Tools Will Never

Dismantle the Master's House," she writes, "Those of us who stand outside the circle of this society's definition of acceptable women; those of us who have been forged in the crucibles of difference—those of us who are poor, who are lesbians, who are Black, who are older—know that survival is not an academic skill. It is learning how to stand alone, unpopular and sometimes reviled, and *how to make common cause with those others identified as outside the structures in order to define and seek a world in which we can all flourish*" (Lorde 1984, 112, emphasis added). I believe Lorde's insight—that true survival for marginalized people requires both self-care and collective action to produce a world in which we can all flourish—is the guidance we need to deal with the contradictory realities of our present world. Cherrie Moraga suggests that Third World feminism is about "feeding people in all their hungers" (Moraga 2000, 130). We can pursue medical and other individualized interventions to alleviate personal suffering and to make our minds/bodies more livable, but only if we make common cause in order to define and seek a more just world will we ever be able to feed people in *all* their hungers.

Acknowledgments

It takes a village to write a book. I would like to express my sincere thanks to my village, especially my family, including my spouse, Daniel Castro; my son, Gabriel Castro-Gupta; my parents, Ann and Satish Gupta; and my dog, Pippi.

I would like to thank all of the faculty, staff, and students involved in the (then named) Department of Women's Studies at Georgetown University and the Department of Women's and Gender Studies at Rutgers University for nurturing me as an undergraduate and master's student.

I first began to think seriously about this project as a doctoral student in women's, gender, and sexuality studies at Emory University. I would like to thank my advisor, Rosemarie Garland-Thomson, for introducing me to the field of disability studies and for always supporting me both professionally and personally. Thank you as well to my other dissertation committee members, Sander Gilman and Mark Risjord. For providing a vibrant interdisciplinary community, thank you to everyone involved with the Emory Center for Mind, Brain, and Culture, especially Robert McCauley and Laura Namy, and to everyone involved with the Emory Neuroethics Program, especially Karen Rommelfanger. Thank you to all of my fellow doctoral students, who provided me with feedback on my work and with fellowship: Harold Braswell, Claire Clark, Amy DeBaets, Megan Friddle, Julia Hass, Nikki Karalekas, Anson Koch-Rein, Jennifer Sarrett, and Kira Walsh. Thanks especially to my queer feminist science studies squad—Cyd Cipolla, David Rubin, and Angie Willey—for supporting me as a graduate student and for remaining my collaborators and friends since graduation. Special thanks to David Rubin for reading and commenting on a complete draft of this manuscript.

I want to thank again the Georgetown Department of Women's Studies, particularly You-Me Park and Leslie Byers, for offering me a job as a visiting assistant professor in the department, for making me feel welcome for the fall semester I was there, for arranging for me to take a full semester of maternity leave in the spring, and for encouraging me to accept a job at Wake Forest University even though my leaving made their own lives more difficult. They consistently put my personal and professional interests above their own.

Thanks as well to all of my colleagues and students in the Department of Women's, Gender, and Sexuality Studies at Wake Forest. A summer writing grant and a semester of pretenure leave were especially helpful in completing this project. I am particularly grateful to the many other assistant professors who have provided friendship, support, and commiseration, particularly the current and former members of my writing group—Elizabeth Clendinning, Amanda Gengler, Stephanie Koscak, Mir Yarfitz, and Nick Albertson. I am also grateful to my other wonderful colleagues, Tanisha Ramachandran, Michaelle Browers, Jarrod Whitaker, Simone Caron, Steve Boyd, Angela Mazaris, and many more. Special thanks to Melissa Jenkins for providing feedback on a draft of this manuscript, among many other things.

I would also like to acknowledge the wonderful community of asexuality studies scholars, who have turned this small subfield into a vibrant and productive space, especially Eunjung Kim, KJ Cerankowski, Ela Przybylo, and Ianna Hawkins Owens, and to the asexually identified individuals who participated in the qualitative research study that I conducted for my dissertation.

Finally, I would like to thank Rutgers University Press, especially editor Kimberly Guinta, for giving me this opportunity and shepherding a first-time author through this process. Thanks to artist Leah Samuels for allowing me to use her artwork for the cover of the book. Genuine thanks as well to the two anonymous reviewers who engaged generously with the manuscript and whose comments helped me improve the manuscript significantly.

Notes

CHAPTER 1 — INTRODUCTION

1. This issue is discussed in detail in the chapter on sexuopharmaceuticals.

2. Examples include physician-assisted suicide (S. M. Wolf 1996; D. Raymond 1999), elective cesarean sections (Beckett 2005; Andrist 2008; Bergeron 2007; Roth and Henley 2012), depression and antidepressants (Fullagar 2009; Gammell and Stoppard 1999; MacKay and Rutherford 2012; Stoppard 2014; Ussher 2010; E. A. Wilson 2006, 2015), and medical interventions into domestic violence (Hurley 2010; Sugg and Inui 1992; Rothenberg 2003; Kurz 1987; Sweet 2014; Tower 2007), among others.

3. Again, the argument does not end here. Bell points out that as a result of these limitations, low-income women are sometimes led to pursue nonnormative forms of motherhood—through formal or informal adoption, for example (Bell 2009). One could therefore make the argument that it is not a bad thing that low-income women have less access to fertility treatments as they are then encouraged, out of necessity, to pursue nonnormative forms of parenting. Indeed, as seen in Chapter 4, some scholars have argued that a lack of access to Viagra is a good thing because it encourages men, out of necessity, to pursue nonnormative forms of sexual pleasure. However, as I argue in Chapter 4, this argument certainly runs the risk of paternalism.

4. Critical analysis tends to be most successful at revealing the power at work in any particular situation but less successful in offering suggestions for what to do. Perhaps conversations about what to do are outside the realm of scholarly inquiry, as they are more conversations about values than about facts (although, of course, facts are also value laden and values can be fact driven). Perhaps this would be a better book if I were to stick to an analysis of *what is*. However, I think I am too much of an activist at heart not to venture into the realm of *what should be*.

5. This argument may call to mind philosophical discussions about "undecidability," particularly in the work of Derrida. Derrida's work suggests that any for/against binary is a false binary, as one side of the binary will always be haunted by the other. From a Derridian perspective, then, our decision between two positions arises not out of epistemic clarity or positive knowledge but out of its lack—thus, undecidability. It is when we do not know what to do, when there is no program or model to follow, when we are

faced with the ethical conundrum of the decision—we have to take a leap of faith (see Derrida 1996, 1999, 2006; for a discussion of the ethics of undecidability, see the conclusion of D. A. Rubin 2017).

6. I use the term "communities of choice" to indicate that people are not atomistic, independent rational choice actors but rather are interdependent with other people, nonhuman animals, and even inanimate objects (for a discussion of relationships with inanimate objects, see M. Y. Chen 2012). I imagine that a person's community of choice might include family, friends, members of relevant identity or political groups, and so on. I do not mean to romanticize the idea of community here—communities can be sites of conflict and inequality. In terms of medical decision making, ethicists insist on the importance of "informed consent"—in other words, patients must be able to make choices about medical interventions based on accurate and comprehensive information. Traditional models of informed consent have tended to assume that patients are independent decision makers. However, some scholars have developed accounts of informed consent that understand humans as relational and emotional (in addition to rational) beings (e.g., Maclean 2013; Lomelino 2015; Fisher 2013; Kluge 2005). These accounts of informed consent suggest how the abstract notion of "individuals deciding in consultation with their communities of choice" could play out in practice.

7. The situation is even more complicated when we consider the situation of those who may not have "normal" decision-making capacities, due to youth, age, or mental disability. There is a substantial literature on this issue by bioethicists and critiques of this literature by scholars within disability studies. To engage with this literature is beyond the scope of this project; overviews are offered in Manson and O'Neill (2007), Maclean (2013), and Lomelino (2015). As already noted, in general, I prefer accounts of informed consent that understand humans as relational and emotional (in addition to rational) beings (e.g., Maclean 2013; Lomelino 2015; Fisher 2013; Kluge 2005).

8. The concept of feminist democratic decision making is explored in the Conclusion to this book.

9. This is exactly the argument made by the reproductive justice movement (D. E. Roberts 2015).

10. I specifically do not use the language of "well-being" or "quality of life" as they are too dependent on concepts of "health." I initially began to use the term "flourishing" alone but found that it too was closely connected to the terms "health," "growth," and "prosperity." A number of scholars, particularly in positive psychology and business, also use the Aristotelian term "eudaimonia" to refer to well-being, quality of life, or human flourishing. However, the meanings of this term in Aristotle's thought are complicated (Capuccino 2015) and their uptake by psychologists and in the field of business has been concerning (Woolfolk and Wasserman 2005). My own university, Wake Forest University, accepted a multimillion-dollar donation from the Koch foundation to start a Eudaimonia Institute, dedicated to the "study of human flourishing" as a strategy to promote libertarian values (Mayer 2016). Recognizing that no term is perfect or resistant to cooptation, I sometimes use the language of "flourishing," sometimes "livability," and sometimes "fulfillment." There are significant bodies of literature in ethics, political philosophy, and moral psychology, among other fields, on what constitutes "well-being." It is beyond the scope of this book to summarize these bodies of literature. For an overview, see Fletcher (2016). In this book, I suggest that individuals, in consultation with their communities of choice, must ultimately be the ones to make the decision about whether

a particular medical intervention is necessary for their well-being. At the same time, I argue that we will need to use feminist democratic processes to decide what type of interventions would promote communal flourishing. It is also my argument that philosophers and moral psychologists will have as much a role to play in making these decisions as scientists, doctors, and other medical professionals.

11. The work in this book is also consonant with much of the work conducted under the rubric of "somatechnics" (Murray and Sullivan 2012). According to Niki Sullivan, the term "somatechnics" is intended to convey "the inextricability of soma and techné, of the body (as a culturally intelligible construct) and the techniques (dispositifs and hard technologies) in and through which corporealities are formed and transformed" (Sullivan 2014, 187). Certainly, in this book, I take the position that soma and techne are inextricable. However, Sullivan describes her work as "deconstructive" and is less interested in adjudicating whether a particular technology should be supported or opposed but in mapping the creation and effects of technological categories and interventions (Sullivan 2014). This is certainly an ethical and political project; as Butler argues, it is an ethical/political project to interrogate the foundations of our thinking (Butler 2013a, 2013b). However, in this project, in addition to engaging in a deconstructive reading, I am also interested in grappling with the issue of what position academics and activists (on the ground so to speak) should take in regards to medical interventions. I believe this focus differentiates this project somewhat from the somatechnics work.

12. I view the type of naturalcultural approach described by Haraway and Barad as a particular kind of social constructionism. Theories about the social construction of gender have always sought to understand the relationship between the biological and the social. To oversimplify, early theories about the social construction of gender often assumed that social differences between the categories of men and women were overlaid on biological differences between males and females. Postmodern approaches to the social construction of gender, exemplified by Judith Butler's theory of gender performativity, have argued that biological differences between males and females are materialized through the repeated "doing" of gender and become visible through an interpretive grid given to us by the heterosexual matrix. Phenomenological approaches and feminist science studies approaches to the social construction of gender take a slightly different approach, arguing that the biological and the social are in constant, iterative "intraaction." Many feminist science studies scholars use the compound term "sex/gender" to indicate that the biological and the social are never separate (Lorber 1994; Butler 1990; I. M. Young 2005; Haraway 1997; Barad 2007).

13. Medical sociologists often use the term "disease" to describe a biological dysfunction and the term "illness" to describe a person's experience of being "sick" in a social context (Conrad and Barker 2010); however, the use of these terms in this way is specific to certain disciplines, and I generally do not use the terms in this way in this book. Rather, I often use the terms "disease" and "illness" interchangeably.

CHAPTER 2 — FEMINIST CRITIQUES OF MEDICINE (AND SOME RESPONSES)

1. "Medically unexplained symptoms" is a medical term for symptoms for which no pathological basis has been determined by the medical profession. Living with symptoms without a medical explanation or diagnosis can have serious consequences, including a lack of social support and a lack of access to needed resources (Nettleton 2006).

2. Public health represents an interesting case, as some public health practitioners focus on larger-scale political and institutional change, while others focus on individual behavior change. Most of the critiques directed against the medical model could be directed against those in public health who focus on individual behavior change through, for example, "health promotion campaigns" (Daykin and Naidoo 1995).

3. Critics also argue that little of the funding raised by these efforts is used to address the environmental causes of breast cancer and that some of the companies that use breast cancer campaigns to market their products simultaneously produce carcinogenic products ("Think Before You Pink" n.d.).

4. The "need" for abortion in the case of fetal anomalies is often cited by prochoice activists as a reason for maintaining abortion access, much to the consternation of some feminist disability studies scholars. As a result, some prolife activists have campaigned against abortion in the case of fetal anomalies, creating a strange potential alliance between disability rights activists and prolife activists (Hubbard 2013). Developing coalitions between disability rights activists and feminist abortion rights activists is necessary to produce a more radical feminist reproductive justice movement.

CHAPTER 3 — THEORIZING FROM TRANSITION-RELATED CARE

1. In the United States, it is illegal for unlicensed practitioners to provide silicone injections. Licensed medical providers may legally offer silicone injections to augment soft tissue, but this usage of silicone injections is not approved by the Food and Drug Administration, and most licensed medical practitioners will not offer liquid silicone injections due to the risk of complication. Rather, to augment soft tissue, U.S. medical practitioners usually inject fat tissue from the patient's own body or use silicone implants, as the plastic pouch around the silicone prevents the silicone from migrating to other parts of the body (Styperek et al. 2013; Rabiner 2012; Medical Board of California 2007).

2. Scholars have analyzed the phenomenon of unlicensed injections of silicone in other contexts; for example, Kulick (1998) discusses this issue in the context of contemporary Brazil. Many thanks to Mir Yarfitz for bringing this scholarship to my attention.

3. There is, of course, a long history of white supremacists equating large buttocks with both women of color and animality (e.g., in the case of Sartjee Baartman), and there is a significant body of excellent feminist scholarship on this topic (e.g., Crais and Scully 2009; Magubane 2001; Sastre 2014; Burns-Ardolino 2009; Beltran 2002).

4. David Valentine rightly critiques the focus of "nontranssexual" feminists and queer theorists on debating the ethics of sex-reassignment surgery (SRS) for transsexual individuals as an exceptional phenomenon, which serves to naturalize the "nontranssexual" body/identity. He suggests that nontranssexual feminists and queer theorists should "frame the desire not to have SRS as a desire and as an act of agency" in order to facilitate viewing this desire "as a desire to hold onto the sexed and gendered meanings that accrete to non-transsexual bodies" (Valentine 2012, 207).

5. It is beyond the scope of this chapter to discuss "detransitioning" or "retransitioning" in depth, but I firmly believe that the same arguments that apply to "transitioning" would apply to "detransitioning" as well.

6. For a discussion of the effects of the revised Gender Identity Disorder / Gender Dysphoria (GID / GD) category on intersex individuals/individuals with "Disorders of Sex Development," see Kraus (2015).

7. Citing the case of an intersex man, Hale Hawbecker, whose male friend did not know Hawbecker did not have testicles, Iain Morland points out that it may be a myth that men necessarily examine each other's genitals in the locker room. Morland argues that in most contexts, it is not "actual" genitals but an assumption about genitals or "cultural genitals" that mean gender. Morland also suggests that the genitals imagined by surgeons are "nostalgic genitals"—phantasmal sites of nostalgia for what never was (Morland 2001).

8. Connections and disconnections between the concepts of "transsexualism" and "paraphilia" in the work of John Money are discussed in Downing, Morland, and Sullivan (2014).

9. The question of restricting access to public bathrooms for transgender people has gained political traction in recent years in the United States, with social conservatives attempting (and in some cases, succeeding) in passing state laws requiring people to use the bathroom that "corresponds with his or her birth sex" (Drum 2016).

10. See also Awkward-Rich (2017) as an example of trans studies scholarship that draws on disability studies as inspiration for the recognition of pain.

11. David Rubin (2015) makes a similar argument in regards to intersex experiences.

12. Of course, many of the procedures that cisgender people access to affirm their gender (such as breast augmentation, liposuction, cosmetic surgery, etc.) have been hotly debated and critiqued by feminist scholars, in a literature referenced in the introduction to this book. The ICATH model does not address the feminist critiques of gender-affirming medical care for cisgender people (particularly ciswomen).

13. The model proposed by ICATH for transition-related care bears some similarity to the "patient-centered care" model embraced by some intersex activists. For a discussion, see D. A. Rubin (2017).

14. A number of scholars have analyzed the intersection of trans issues with capitalism. One of the arguments for granting trans people access to transition-related care has long been that such care will allow trans people to become productive, working members of society (Irving 2008). In addition, scholars and activists have pointed out that transition-related care can be profit-generating for those providing it—from doctors and mental health professionals to pharmaceutical companies to those who arrange for Western individuals to travel to places like Bangkok in order to obtain "gender reassignment surgery" (O'Brien 2013; Aizura 2009, 2010; David 2017). Changing the way transition-related care is delivered would certainly alter some of the capitalist relations currently involved.

15. Toby Beauchamp argues that in addition to reflecting fears about athletes "doping," the classification of testosterone as a controlled substance reflected fears of gender nonconformity and racialized fears about porous national boundaries and the degeneration of the national body (Beauchamp 2013; see also Gill-Peterson 2014).

16. While Loretta Ross (who coined the term "reproductive justice" and has been a leader in the reproductive justice movement) very much frames this movement in terms of an international human rights framework, there may be other articulations of reproductive justice that do not rely on a human rights framework. For example, it may be possible to use only the language of "justice" in place of the language of rights.

CHAPTER 4 — SEXUOPHARMACEUTICALS

1. The letter is available online at http://www.scribd.com/doc/205503946/Group-Letter
-Supporting-Treatment-for-Female-Sexual-Dysfunction (accessed October 2, 2014). The

press release is available online at http://www.prnewswire.com/news-releases/national
-consumers-league-and-now—fda-delays-approval-of-first-ever-drug-treatment-for
-low-sexual-desire-in-women-244888421.html (accessed October 2, 2014).

2. Viagra was originally tested as a treatment for heart disease. In more detail, Viagra works by inhibiting phosphodiesterase type 5 (PDE5). Inhibiting PDE5 enhances the effects of nitric oxide (NO). NO, in turn, activates an enzyme that results in increased levels of cyclic guanosine monophosphate (cGMP). cGMP causes muscle relaxation in the penis, which allows for an inflow of blood into the penis. Thus, when sexual stimulation causes a localized increase of NO, the inhibition of PDE5 by Viagra causes increased levels of cGMP, which allows blood to flow into the penis, leading to an erection (Padma-Nathan 2006).

3. Of course, it is important to critically analyze questionnaires such as the Female Sexual Function Index in order to see how they are measuring female sexual satisfaction (see Flore 2013, 2014).

4. In some of the scholarship on Viagra, it is sometimes difficult to tell whether the scholar is critiquing what I call the broader discursive formation of Viagra (which includes media depictions of Viagra, Viagra ads, medical education related to Viagra, etc.) and the way Viagra as a drug is used by actual people. Although both "Viagra the discursive formation" and "Viagra the drug" are material-semiotic phenomena and are intrarelated, they are not the same material-semiotic phenomenon. I hazard that this confusing use of language is either reflective of or contributes to the difficulty some critical theorists have in recognizing that there might be differences between how a drug is conceptualized and marketed by its creators and how it is understood and used by individuals.

5. Kerner first began experimenting with cunnilingus as a result of sexual difficulties. He soon embraced cunnilingus as a core sexuality activity. In his 2004 book, *She Comes First: The Thinking Man's Guide to Pleasuring a Woman*, he challenges the societal privileging of penile-vaginal intercourse and urges his male readers to embrace oral sex in order to create a shared experience of pleasure, writing, "It's time to close the sex gap and create a level playing field in the exchange of pleasure, and cunnilingus is far more than just a means for achieving this noble end; it's the cornerstone of a new sexual paradigm, one that exuberantly extols a shared experience of pleasure, intimacy, respect, and contentment" (Kerner 2004, 4).

6. Although I agree with much of Baglia's argument, I find problematic his implied suggestion that men should be "forced" to experiment sexually as a result of impotence. In addition, there is the possibility that Viagra itself could be considered a form of sexual experimentation, albeit a highly regulated and regulatory one. People who seek out Viagra may be (perhaps unconsciously) experimenting with what bio/psycho pharmaceuticals do to their bodies and also what their bodies do to pharmaceuticals (see E. A. Wilson 2015). Thank you to David Rubin for this later insight.

7. In *Testo Junkie*, Paul Preciado argues that Viagra is part of what he calls a pharmacopornographic regime, in which drug companies and the pornographic industry produce sexual subjectivities and desires that can be transformed into capital—pleasure capital. For Preciado then, drugs like Viagra form a key part of biopolitical control. Preciado also experiments with using drugs (in his case, testosterone gel) in ways contrary to the demands of the pharmacopornographic regime (Preciado 2013).

8. As another example, in *Testo Junkie*, Paul Preciado describes the ways in which self-administering testosterone gel facilitates his experiences of sexual pleasure (Preciado 2013). See previous endnote.

9. In addition, minor changes were made to the definitions and criteria in each category, and subjective personal distress was retained as a criterion for most of the categories. A new diagnosis of noncoital sexual pain disorder was added to the category of sexual pain disorders. In addition, members of the conference proposed adding a category called sexual satisfaction disorder, to apply to women who are "unable to achieve subjective sexual satisfaction, despite adequate desire, arousal and orgasm" (Basson et al. 2000, 892), but this category was not adopted by the conference (Basson et al. 2000).

10. All of the women in this study were diagnosed with the umbrella diagnosis of female sexual dysfunction (FSD) and with the more specific diagnosis of female sexual arousal disorder (FSAD), but only 40 to 50 percent of the women had a primary diagnosis of FSAD. Even the women with primary diagnoses of FSAD usually had some other specific sexual dysfunction as well, as FSAD rarely appears in isolation in women. In this study, no significant difference was found between Viagra and the placebo in improving measures of sexual function and satisfaction, although there was a strong placebo effect (Basson et al. 2002).

11. One such study found that Viagra was effective for some women with FSAD related to the use of selective serotonin reuptake inhibitors (SSRIs) (a class of antidepressants) (Nurnberg et al. 2008).

12. Two primary studies, each enrolling around 500 participants, were used to evaluate the effectiveness of Intrinsa. In the first study, participants using Instrinsa reported around two additional sexually satisfying events per month (the primary study end point), while participants using the placebo reported around one additional sexually satisfying event per month. The second study had similar results. In both studies, participants using Intrinsa also scored higher on a measure of sexual desire than at baseline (and the increase was about 5 points greater on a 100-point scale than for those receiving the placebo) and lower on a measure of sexual distress than at baseline (and the decrease was about 6–7 points greater on a 100-point scale than for those receiving the placebo) (D. Davis 2004). In both studies, participants using Instrinsa also reported the following benefits (again, to a slightly greater extent than the participants receiving the placebo): arousal, orgasm, improvement in sexual pleasure, reduction of sexual concerns, improved sexual responsiveness, and improved sexual self-image (J. D. Lucas 2004). Of the participants receiving Intrinsa, 52 percent felt they had a meaningful benefit, while 31 percent of the participants receiving the placebo felt they had a meaningful benefit (D. Davis 2004).

13. The fear of "side effects" such as hirsutism may reflect a fear of gender nonconformity, the "masculinization" of women, and transphobia. There is a need for further research into the connection between hormone therapy for transgender individuals and Intrinsa, as research on the former was used at the FDA hearing on Intrinsa (Food and Drug Administration [FDA] 2004). For a discussion of testosterone regulation from a trans studies perspective, see Beauchamp (2012) and Gill-Peterson (2014).

14. A prop designer has a number of advertisements for flibanserin included in her online portfolio, and she states that the ads were created for Boehringer Ingelheim. The ads are available here: http://www.lizengelhardt.com/props/ad-fibancerin (accessed November 2, 2013).

15. Again, see: http://www.lizengelhardt.com/props/ad-fibancerin (accessed November 2, 2013).

16. This section comes from Gupta (2013b, 2015b).

17. The *DSM-IV-TR* included the diagnosis of hypoactive sexual desire disorder (HSDD), which was defined as "persistently or recurrently deficient or absent sexual fantasies and desire for sexual activity," which must have caused "marked distress or interpersonal difficulty" (Brotto 2010). For the *DSM-5*, released in 2013, HSDD was restricted to apply to men only and a combined category called "sexual interest/arousal disorder" was created for women to reflect the results of research showing that sexual interest and sexual arousal are not necessarily separate stages for women (American Psychiatric Association 2013; for some of the reasoning behind this change, see Basson 2000; for a critique of this reasoning, see Tyler 2008). However, because contemporary asexual activism and scholarship on contemporary asexualities have focused on the *DSM-IV-TR*, I focus on the definition of HSDD in the *DSM-IV-TR* in this chapter.

18. The report is not public. I was given access to a redacted version of the report by the authors of the report. For more, see a blog post by one of the report's authors (Hinderliter 2009).

19. Other formulations by asexually identified people use the more gender-inclusive terminology "attraction to neither males nor females nor people of other genders."

20. Suggestions made by asexual activists do seem to have been incorporated into the *DSM* revision process. For the *DMS-5*, the category of HSDD was retained for men and a separate category—female sexual interest/arousal disorder—was created for women. For both diagnoses, the accompanying text indicates that a "desire discrepancy," in which a person has lower desire for sexual activity than their partner, is not sufficient for a diagnosis. In addition, for both diagnoses, the text indicates that if a person's low desire is explained by self-identification as an "asexual," then a diagnosis should not be made (American Psychiatric Association 2013).

21. For a description of this research, see Gupta (2017).

CHAPTER 5 — CONSTRUCTING FAT, CONSTRUCTING FAT STIGMA

1. Of course, the line between individual-level and population-level interventions is not a hard and fast one. In addition, there have certainly been people who have argued that "gender dysphoria"/transition-related care (e.g., Rotondi et al. 2013) and sexual dissatisfaction/sexual enhancement interventions (e.g., Laumann, Paik, and Rosen 1999) should be seen as public health issues, but compared to "obesity"/weight-loss interventions, there is much less public health discourse in regards to these two issues.

2. Even the mainstream left expressed some discomfort with Obama when she referenced her own daughters' weights in a speech about the campaign (Khan 2010).

3. Practices like feederism—in which one derives sexual pleasure from eating/being fed and/or feeding others—are certainly rendered unintelligible by this moral logic (for analyses of feederism, see Giovanelli and Peluso 2006; Charles and Palkowski 2015).

4. For example, the National Organization for Women (NOW) celebrated "Love Your Body Day" on October 14, 2014 (http://now.org/now-foundation/love-your-body/).

5. For example, activism against an advertising campaign by Protein World in the London Underground featuring a skinny, bikini-clad model next to the tagline "Are you beach body ready?" led the United Kingdom's Advertising Standards Authority (ASA) to pull the advertisements (Crocker 2015). Twitter campaigns like #BraveGirlsWant and #TruthInAds (from the Brave Girls Alliance) and #NotBuyingIt and #MediaWeLike (from the Representation Project) have called out various forms of sexism in advertising. Activists supported the introduction of a bill to the U.S. Congress (called the

"Truth in Advertising" act) that would require the U.S. Federal Trade Commission (FTC) to investigate the use of images in advertising that "have been altered to materially change the physical characteristics of the faces and bodies of the individuals depicted" (Cunningham 2014; C. Dewey 2014). *Ms. Magazine* has long featured a "no comment" section that calls out questionable advertising (see http://msmagazine.com/nocommentarchive.asp).

6. Examples include a social media campaign with the hashtag "fatkini" featuring fat women taking selfies in their swimsuits (Fischer 2015) and "The Adipositivity Project," a collection of photographs featuring "fat physicality" (http://adipositivity.com/).

7. What exactly is involved in these "support" or "intervention" groups is not always clear from the published literature, an issue deserving of further attention.

8. It may be entirely possible that one's internal cues might lead one to eat in a nonnormative or even supposedly "unhealthy" way.

9. Many thanks to David Rubin for this insight.

10. A number of feminist scholars have argued that it is a mistake to view socially produced differences as easily changeable but biological differences as unchangeable bedrock (Grosz 1990; Kirby 1991).

11. However, Ernsberger argues that fat is not a consequence of poverty but rather is the cause of poverty as fat people are discriminated against in employment (Ernsberger 2009). Yancey, Leslie, and Abel (2006) make a somewhat similar argument to the one I am making here, calling on feminists to take the health consequences of weight seriously and to recognize the ways in which structural factors lead to higher levels of fatness among socially marginalized groups. However, their argument is one-sided, suggesting that feminists adopt public health approaches, rather than arguing that feminist and public health approaches are both limited but could be combined, and they do not take a disability studies approach to the issue or question the pursuit of health as a worthy goal (Yancey, Leslie, and Abel 2006).

12. Certainly, what counts as "healthy" or "nutritious" food and a "healthy" or "nutritious" diet is worthy of interrogation. The U.S. Department of Health and Human Services and the U.S. Department of Agriculture's dietary guidelines for 2015–2020 recommend limiting calories to a certain level based on age, sex/gender, and level of physical activity and eating a diet that generally includes vegetables, fruits, grains (especially whole grains), fat-free or low-fat dairy (which includes soy), proteins, and oils, while limiting consumption of saturated and *trans* fats, added sugars, and sodium. Of course, what counts as a "healthy" diet will differ for people with certain "health conditions," for pregnant people, and so on (U.S. Department of Health and Human Services and U.S. Department of Agriculture 2015). In addition, as discussed later in this chapter, I argue that whether a particular eating pattern is healthy for an individual must be determined based on the entire context of a person's life—perhaps someone eats a diet high in saturated and *trans* fats because to find other foods would cause significant stress, and the negative health impact of added stress would be greater than the negative health impact of eating high levels of saturated and *trans* fats. Or perhaps a person eats a diet high in added sugars because this particular diet allows this person to strengthen relations with a particular community of people, and the health benefits that accrue from this social support network are greater than the health damages that accrue from the added sugar.

13. Scholars in black studies such as Saidyia Hartman and Fred Moten suggest that we cannot think corporeality outside of history, including the history of antiblackness. Thus,

the comparatively higher rates of "fatness" among black women cannot be dissociated from the history of antiblackness dating back to the transatlantic slave trade and chattel slavery (Hartman 1997; Moten 2017; Sexton 2008). Thanks to David Rubin for this insight.

14. The public health approach to obesity often models itself after the public health approach to smoking, which involves both "individualist" campaigns to educate the public about the health effects of smoking as well as more "collective" campaigns such as outlawing the advertisement of cigarettes to children, banning smoking in public buildings, and leveling high taxes on cigarette consumption. The public health campaign against smoking has been, by some metrics, remarkably successful, as overall rates of smoking have decreased significantly and smoking, particularly in public, is now a stigmatized activity. However, analysts have questioned whether stigmatizing people who are addicted to nicotine is helpful or hurtful, whether economically and socially marginalized individuals have the resources required to quit, and whether quitting smoking is necessarily the best option for individuals who smoke as a form of self-medication (T. Brown, Platt, and Amos 2014; Niederdeppe et al. 2008; Thompson, Barnett, and Pearce 2009; Kumari and Postma 2005; Daykin and Naidoo 1995; Oaks 2001).

15. See footnote 12.

16. The term "choice architecture" was invented or popularized by Richard Thaler and Cass Sunstein in their 2008 book *Nudge: Improving Decisions about Health, Wealth, and Happiness*. It describes a general effort to create an environment in which individuals are "nudged" to choose socially desirable behaviors (Thaler and Sunstein 2009).

17. I would go so far as to argue that people may find pleasure and/or "flourishing" (not necessarily the same thing) in "self-destruction." This argument bears some relationship to psychoanalytic arguments about the "death drive" and the way these arguments have been taken up in queer theory as the "antisocial thesis" (for a recent discussion of the antisocial thesis in queer theory, see Wiegman 2017). A number of queer/fat studies scholars have argued that antiobesity discourses rely on a celebration of the "reproductive futurity" critiqued by Lee Edelman in *No Future: Queer Theory and the Death Drive* (2004). These scholars have also highlighted examples of fat activism that refuse redemptive models of fatness. Francis Ray White argues, for example, that embracing a "future-negating politics" may open up "the possibility of multiple queer futures for fat which, despite their apparent anti-sociality, may in fact offer some of us more of a life" (White 2012, 15; see also Chalklin 2016).

18. There may be particular moral reasons for some individuals to eat nutritious food and/or engage in physical activity. For example, those who provide care for dependents may feel some obligation to engage in life-prolonging activities in order to be able to continue to provide care for their dependents. However, these moral obligations are not universal.

19. Orlistat, in particular, is known for its gastrointestinal side effects like "fatty/oily stool, faecal urgency, and oily spotting" (Rucker et al. 2007).

20. There is some evidence that bariatric surgeries actually work by altering the microbial community of the body (Furet et al. 2010; Kong et al. 2013; Zhang et al. 2009), suggesting that Elizabeth Wilson's analysis of the gut in *Gut Feminism* may have some relevance to this discussion, although I do not have the space to explore these connections (E. A. Wilson 2015).

21. The percentage of excess weight loss (EWL) is generally calculated as follows: percent EWL = 100 percent × (weight lost) ÷ (preoperative weight − ideal body weight [IBW])

(Obeidat et al. 2015). Of course, this definition/calculation reflects value judgments and is open to critique.

22. Indeed, many of the feminists who have critiqued the culture that contributes to the production of eating-disordered behavior have argued that it can still be appropriate to treat anorexia through medical interventions (see, e.g., Bordo 2004). While this is not exactly analogous to the case of acute heaviness, the comparison is worth considering.

23. Research has demonstrated that among those who are considered "medically eligible" for bariatric surgery, minority individuals and low-income individuals are less likely to undergo bariatric surgery (M. Martin et al. 2010; Wallace et al. 2010); however, as argued in this chapter, minority and low-income individuals also have less access to the medical interventions of diet and exercise.

CHAPTER 6 — CONCLUSION

1. Again, there are significant bodies of literature in ethics, political philosophy, and moral psychology, among other fields, on what constitutes "well-being." It is beyond the scope of this book to summarize these bodies of literature. For an overview, see Fletcher (2016).

2. The Nazis used the phrase "life unworthy of life" or "lives not worth living" to designate groups of people—like people with disabilities—that, in Nazi thinking, had no right to live and were the proper targets of euthanasia programs (Proctor 1988; Friedlander 1997). The question "who has the right to determine who should and who should not inhabit the world" comes from Ruth Hubbard's rephrasing of Hannah Arendt (Hubbard 2013).

References

Adler, Nancy E., and Katherine Newman. 2002. "Socioeconomic Disparities in Health: Pathways and Policies." *Health Affairs (Project Hope)* 21 (2): 60–76.

African American Policy Forum. n.d. *A Primer on Intersectionality.* New York: African American Policy Forum.

Ahmed, Sara. 2006. *Queer Phenomenology: Orientations, Objects, Others.* Durham, NC: Duke University Press.

Aizura, Aren Z. 2009. "Where Health and Beauty Meet: Femininity and Racialisation in Thai Cosmetic Surgery Clinics." *Asian Studies Review* 33 (3): 303–317.

———. 2010. "Feminine Transformations: Gender Reassignment Surgical Tourism in Thailand." *Medical Anthropology* 29 (4): 424–443.

Albertson Fineman, Martha. 2008. "The Vulnerable Subject: Anchoring Equality in the Human Condition." *Yale Journal of Law and Feminism* 20: 1.

Alcoff, Linda. 1993. *Feminist Epistemologies.* New York: Routledge.

Alexander-Floyd, Nikol G. 2012. "Disappearing Acts: Reclaiming Intersectionality in the Social Sciences in a Post-Black Feminist Era." *Feminist Formations* 24 (1): 1–25.

American Psychiatric Association. 1980. *Diagnostic and Statistical Manual of Mental Disorders.* 3rd ed. Washington, DC: American Psychiatric Association.

———. 2000. *Diagnostic and Statistical Manual of Mental Disorders: DSM-IV-TR.* Washington, DC: American Psychiatric Association.

———. 2013. *Diagnostic and Statistical Manual of Mental Disorders.* 5th ed. Arlington, VA: American Psychiatric Association.

American Public Health Association (APHA). 2007. "Toward a Healthy Sustainable Food System." https://www.apha.org/policies-and-advocacy/public-health-policy-statements/policy-database/2014/07/29/12/34/toward-a-healthy-sustainable-food-system.

Amy, N. K., A. Aalborg, P. Lyons, and L. Keranen. 2005. "Barriers to Routine Gynecological Cancer Screening for White and African-American Obese Women." *International Journal of Obesity* 30 (1): 147–155.

Anderson, Elizabeth. 2004. "Uses of Value Judgments in Science: A General Argument, with Lessons from a Case Study of Feminist Research on Divorce." *Hypatia* 19 (1): 1–24.

Anderson, Karen O., Carmen R. Green, and Richard Payne. 2009. "Racial and Ethnic Disparities in Pain: Causes and Consequences of Unequal Care." *The Journal of Pain* 10 (12): 1187–1204.

Anderson-Minshall, Diane. 2012. "Bogus Doc Had Trans Victims Nationwide." *The Advocate*, January 2, 2012. https://www.advocate.com/news/daily-news/2012/01/02/bogus-doc-had-trans-victims-nationwide.

Andrist, Linda C. 2008. "The Implications of Objectification Theory for Women's Health: Menstrual Suppression and 'Maternal Request' Cesarean Delivery." *Health Care for Women International* 29 (5): 551–565.

Angell, Marcia. 2005. *The Truth about the Drug Companies: How They Deceive Us and What to Do about It*. Reprint ed. New York: Random House Trade Paperbacks.

Angrisani, L., A. Santonicola, P. Iovino, G. Formisano, H. Buchwald, and N. Scopinaro. 2015. "Bariatric Surgery Worldwide 2013." *Obesity Surgery* 25 (10): 1822–1832.

"Anyone Have Luck Getting Electrolysis Covered by Insurance?" n.d. *Reddit Asktransgender*. Accessed April 18, 2017. https://www.reddit.com/r/asktransgender/comments/4ebe1a/anyone_have_luck_getting_electrolysis_covered_by/.

Apovian, Caroline M., Louis J. Aronne, Daniel H. Bessesen, Marie E. McDonnell, M. Hassan Murad, Uberto Pagotto, Donna H. Ryan, Christopher D. Still, and Endocrine Society. 2015. "Pharmacological Management of Obesity: An Endocrine Society Clinical Practice Guideline." *Journal of Clinical Endocrinology and Metabolism* 100 (2): 342–362.

Asexual Visibility and Education Network. n.d. "Overview." Accessed October 18, 2013. http://www.asexuality.org/home/overview.html.

Association for Size Diversity and Health. 2010. "ASDAH Letter to Michelle Obama." February 9. https://www.sizediversityandhealth.org/content.asp?id=205&articleID=75.

Athanasiou, Thanos, Vanash Patel, George Garas, Hutan Ashrafian, Louise Hull, Nick Sevdalis, Sian Harding, Ara Darzi, and Sotirios Paroutis. 2016. "Mentoring Perception, Scientific Collaboration and Research Performance: Is There a 'Gender Gap' in Academic Medicine? An Academic Health Science Centre Perspective." *Postgraduate Medical Journal* 92 (1092): 581–586.

Awkward-Rich, Cameron. 2017. "Trans, Feminism: Or, Reading Like a Depressed Transsexual." *Signs: Journal of Women in Culture and Society* 42 (4): 819–841.

Bacon, Linda, and Lucy Aphramor. 2011. "Weight Science: Evaluating the Evidence for a Paradigm Shift." *Nutrition Journal* 10: 9.

Baglia, Jay. 2005. *The Viagra Ad Venture: Masculinity, Marketing, and the Performance of Sexual Health*. New York: Peter Lang.

Ballantyne, Garth H. 2003. "Measuring Outcomes Following Bariatric Surgery: Weight Loss Parameters, Improvement in Co-Morbid Conditions, Change in Quality of Life and Patient Satisfaction." *Obesity Surgery* 13 (6): 954–964.

Balsa, Ana I., and Thomas G. McGuire. 2003. "Prejudice, Clinical Uncertainty and Stereotyping as Sources of Health Disparities." *Journal of Health Economics* 22 (1): 89–116.

Barad, Karen. 2007. *Meeting the Universe Halfway: Quantum Physics and the Entanglement of Matter and Meaning*. Durham, NC: Duke University Press Books.

"Bariatric Surgery Side Effects." n.d. The National Institute of Diabetes and Digestive and Kidney Diseases. Accessed February 22, 2017. https://www.niddk.nih.gov

/health-information/health-topics/weight-control/bariatric-surgery/Pages/side
-effects.aspx.

Baril, Alexandre. 2015. "Transness as Debility: Rethinking Intersections between Trans and Disabled Embodiments." *Feminist Review* 111 (1): 59–74.

Basson, Rosemary. 2000. "The Female Sexual Response: A Different Model." *Journal of Sex & Marital Therapy* 26 (1): 51–65.

Basson, Rosemary, Jennifer Berman, Arthur Burnett, Leonard Derogatis, David Ferguson, Jean Fourcroy, Irwin Goldstein, et al. 2000. "Report of the International Consensus Development Conference on Female Sexual Dysfunction: Definitions and Classifications." *The Journal of Urology* 163 (3): 888–893.

Basson, Rosemary, Rosemary McInnes, Mike D. Smith, Gemma Hodgson, and Nandan Koppiker. 2002. "Efficacy and Safety of Sildenafil Citrate in Women with Sexual Dysfunction Associated with Female Sexual Arousal Disorder." *Journal of Women's Health & Gender-Based Medicine* 11 (4): 367–377.

Bayer, Ronald. 1987. *Homosexuality and American Psychiatry*. Princeton, N.J.: Princeton University Press.

Baynton, Douglas C. 2013. "Disability and the Justification of Inequality in American History." In *The Disability Studies Reader*, ed. Lennard Davis, 33–57. New York: Routledge.

Beauchamp, Toby. 2012. "The Substance of Borders: Transgender Politics, Mobility, and US State Regulation of Testosterone." *GLQ: A Journal of Lesbian and Gay Studies* 19 (1): 57–78.

Beckett, Katherine. 2005. "Choosing Cesarean Feminism and the Politics of Childbirth in the United States." *Feminist Theory* 6 (3): 251–275.

Bell, Ann V. 2009. "'It's Way out of My League' Low-Income Women's Experiences of Medicalized Infertility." *Gender & Society* 23 (5): 688–709.

Bella, Anthony J., Jay C. Lee, Serge Carrier, Francois Bénard, and Gerald B. Brock. 2015. "2015 CUA Practice Guidelines for Erectile Dysfunction." *Canadian Urological Association Journal* 9 (1–2): 23–29.

Beltran, Mary. 2002. "The Hollywood Latina Body as Site of Social Struggle: Media Constructions of Stardom and Jennifer Lopez's 'Cross-over Butt.'" *Quarterly Review of Film and Video* 19 (1): 71–86.

Benjamin, Henry. 1996. *The Trasnssexual Phenomenon*. New York: Julian Press.

Bergeron, Veronique. 2007. "The Ethics of Cesarean Section on Maternal Request: A Feminist Critique of the American College of Obstetricians and Gynecologists' Position on Patient-Choice Surgery." *Bioethics* 21 (9): 478–487.

Boorse, Christopher. 1975. "On the Distinction between Disease and Illness." *Philosophy & Public Affairs* 5 (1): 49–68.

Bordo, Susan. 2004. *Unbearable Weight: Feminism, Western Culture, and the Body*. Berkeley: University of California Press.

Bornstein, Kate. 1995. *Gender Outlaw: On Men, Women and the Rest of Us*. Reprint ed. New York: Vintage.

Botz-Bornstein, Thorsten. 2011. "America and Viagra or How the White Negro Became a Little Whiter: Viagra as an Afro-Disiac." In *The Philosophy of Viagra*, ed Thorsten Botz-Bornstein, 145–155. Amsterdam: Rodopi.

Bowen, Sarah, Sinikka Elliott, and Joslyn Brenton. 2014. "The Joy of Cooking?" *Contexts* 13 (3): 20–25.

Brethauer, Stacy A., Bipan Chand, and Philip R. Schauer. 2006. "Risks and Benefits of Bariatric Surgery: Current Evidence." *Cleveland Clinic Journal of Medicine* 73 (11): 993.

Briggs, Laura. 2000. "The Race of Hysteria: 'Overcivilization' and the 'Savage' Woman in Late Nineteenth-Century Obstetrics and Gynecology." *American Quarterly* 52 (2): 246–273.

———. 2002. *Reproducing Empire: Race, Sex, Science, and U.S. Imperialism in Puerto Rico.* Berkeley: University of California Press.

Brotto, Lori A. 2010. "The DSM Diagnostic Criteria for Hypoactive Sexual Desire Disorder in Women." *Archives of Sexual Behavior* 39 (2): 221–239.

Brotto, Lori A., and Morag A. Yule. 2009. "Reply to Hinderliter (2009)." *Archives of Sexual Behavior* 38 (July): 622–623.

———. 2011. "Physiological and Subjective Sexual Arousal in Self-Identified Asexual Women." *Archives of Sexual Behavior* 40 (4): 699–712.

Brown, Anna. 2017. "Transgender Issues Sharply Divide Republicans, Democrats." *Pew Research Center* (blog). November 8, 2017. http://www.pewresearch.org/fact-tank/2017/11/08/transgender-issues-divide-republicans-and-democrats/.

Brown, Tamara, Stephen Platt, and Amanda Amos. 2014. "Equity Impact of Population-Level Interventions and Policies to Reduce Smoking in Adults: A Systematic Review." *Drug and Alcohol Dependence* 138 (Suppl. C): 7–16.

Brudney, Daniel. 2009. "Beyond Autonomy and Best Interests." *Hastings Center Report* 39 (2): 31–37.

Burgard, Deb. 2009. "What Is Health at Every Size." In *The Fat Studies Reader*, ed. Esther Rothblum and Sondra Solovay, 41–53. New York: NYU Press.

Burgard, Deb, Elana Dykewoman, Esther Rothblum, and Pattie Thomas. 2009. "Are We Ready to Throw Our Weight Around? Fat Studies and Political Activism." In *The Fat Studies Reader*, ed. Esther Rothblum and Sondra Solovay, 334–340. New York: NYU Press.

Burke, Mary C. 2011. "Resisting Pathology: GID and the Contested Terrain of Diagnosis in the Transgender Rights Movement." In *Sociology of Diagnosis*, ed. P. J. McGann and David J. Hutson, 183–210. Bingley, UK: Emerald Group Publishing Limited.

Burns-Ardolino, Wendy A. 2009. "Jiggle in My Walk: The Iconic Power of the 'Big Butt' in American Pop Culture." In *The Fat Studies Reader*, ed. Esther Rothblum and Sondra Solovay, 271–279. New York: NYU Press.

Butler, Judith. 1990. *Gender Trouble: Feminism and the Subversion of Identity.* New York: Routledge.

———. 1993. *Bodies That Matter: On the Discursive Limits of Sex.* New York: Routledge.

———. 2004. *Undoing Gender.* New York: Routledge.

———. 2006. *Precarious Life: The Powers of Mourning and Violence.* Reprint ed. London: Verso.

———. 2013a. "Contingent Foundations." In *Feminist Contentions: A Philosophical Exchange*, ed. Judith Butler, Seyla Benhabib, Nancy Fraser, and Drucilla Cornell. New York: Routledge.

———. 2013b. "For a Careful Reading." In *Feminist Contentions: A Philosophical Exchange*, ed. Judith Butler, Seyla Benhabib, Nancy Fraser, and Drucilla Cornell. New York: Routledge.

———. 2016. *Frames of War: When Is Life Grievable?* Reprint ed. London: Verso.

Byne, William, Susan J. Bradley, Eli Coleman, A. Evan Eyler, Richard Green, Edgardo J. Menvielle, Heino F. L. Meyer-Bahlburg, Richard R. Pleak, and D. Andrew Tompkins. 2012. "Report of the American Psychiatric Association Task Force on Treatment of Gender Identity Disorder." *Archives of Sexual Behavior* 41 (4): 759–796.

Campos, Paul. 2004. *The Obesity Myth: Why America's Obsession with Weight Is Hazardous to Your Health*. New York: Gotham.

Capuccino, Carlotta. 2015. "Happiness and Aristotle's Definition of Eudaimonia." *Philosophical Topics* 41 (1): 1–26.

Castañeda, Claudia. 2015. "Developing Gender: The Medical Treatment of Transgender Young People." *Social Science & Medicine* 143 (October): 262–270.

Centers for Disease Control and Prevention (CDC). 2007. "Adult Obesity Causes & Consequences." https://www.cdc.gov/obesity/adult/causes.html.

Chakrabarti, Pratik. 2013. *Medicine and Empire: 1600–1960*. New York: Palgrave Macmillan.

Chalklin, Vikki. 2016. "Obstinate Fatties: Fat Activism, Queer Negativity, and the Celebration of 'Obesity.'" *Subjectivity* 9 (2): 107–125.

Chang, Su-Hsin, Carolyn R. T. Stoll, Jihyun Song, J. Esteban Varela, Christopher J. Eagon, and Graham A. Colditz. 2014. "The Effectiveness and Risks of Bariatric Surgery: An Updated Systematic Review and Meta-Analysis, 2003-2012." *JAMA Surgery* 149 (3): 275–287.

Charles, Kathy, and Michael Palkowski. 2015. *Feederism: Eating, Weight Gain, and Sexual Pleasure*. New York: Palgrave Macmillan.

Chasin, C. J. DeLuzio. 2011. "Theoretical Issues in the Study of Asexuality." *Archives of Sexual Behavior* 40 (4): 713–723.

Chen, Jie, Arturo Vargas-Bustamante, Karoline Mortensen, and Alexander N. Ortega. 2016. "Racial and Ethnic Disparities in Health Care Access and Utilization under the Affordable Care Act." *Medical Care* 54 (2): 140–146.

Chen, Mel Y. 2012. *Animacies: Biopolitics, Racial Mattering, and Queer Affect*. Durham, NC: Duke University Press.

Cho, Sumi, Kimberlé Williams Crenshaw, and Leslie McCall. 2013. "Toward a Field of Intersectionality Studies: Theory, Applications, and Praxis." *Signs* 38 (4): 785–810.

Chrisler, Joan C., and Paula Caplan. 2002. "The Strange Case of Dr. Jekyll and Ms. Hyde: How PMS Became a Cultural Phenomenon and a Psychiatric Disorder." *Annual Review of Sex Research* 13 (1): 274–306.

Clare, Eli. 2017. *Brilliant Imperfection: Grappling with Cure*. Durham, NC: Duke University Press.

Clare, Eli, Dean Spade, and Aurora Levins Morales. 2015. *Exile and Pride: Disability, Queerness, and Liberation*. Reissue ed. Durham, NC: Duke University Press Books.

Clark, Lucian. 2013. "Detransition and Trans Regret." *GenderTerror* (blog). December 13, 2013. https://genderterror.com/2013/12/13/detransition-and-trans-regret/.

Clarke, Adele E., Laura Mamo, Jennifer R. Fishman, Janet K. Shim, and Jennifer Ruth Fosket. 2003. "Biomedicalization: Technoscientifc Transformations of Health Illness and U.S. Biomedicine." *American Sociological Review* 68 (2): 161–194.

Clarke, Toni. 2014. "FDA Hits Back at Charge of Gender Bias in Libido Drug Decision." *Reuters*, February 12, 2014. http://www.reuters.com/article/2014/02/12/us-sprout-fda-idUSBREA1B00B20140212.

Coates, Penelope. 2005. "Androgen Insufficiency in Ageing Men: How Is It Defined and Should It Be Treated?" *Clinical Biochemist Reviews* 26 (1): 37–41.

Coeytaux, Francine, and Victoria Nichols. 2014. "Plan C: The Safe Strategy for a Missed Period When You Don't Want to Be Pregnant." *Rewire*, February 7, 2014. https://rewire .news/article/2014/02/07/plan-c-safe-strategy-missed-period-dont-want-pregnant/.

Cohen, Joshua. 2018. "Female Sex Drive Booster Addyi Is Back, but Will Second Time around Be Different?" *Forbes.com*, June 18, 2018. https://www.forbes.com/sites /joshuacohen/2018/06/18/female-sex-drive-booster-addyi-is-back-but-will-second -time-around-be-different/#7458d4de794d.

Cohen-Kettenis, Peggy T., and Friedemann Pfäfflin. 2009. "The DSM Diagnostic Criteria for Gender Identity Disorder in Adolescents and Adults." *Archives of Sexual Behavior* 39 (2): 499–513.

Collins, Dana, Sylvanna Falcón, Sharmila Lodhia, and Molly Talcott. 2010. "New Directions in Feminism and Human Rights." *International Feminist Journal of Politics* 12 (3–4): 298–318.

Collins, Patricia Hill. 2005. *Black Sexual Politics: African Americans, Gender, and the New Racism*. New ed. New York: Routledge.

Colman, Eric. 2005. "Anorectics on Trial: A Half Century of Federal Regulation of Prescription Appetite Suppressants." *Annals of Internal Medicine* 143 (5): 380.

Conrad, Peter. 1992. "Medicalization and Social Control." *Annual Review of Sociology* 18: 209–232.

———. 1994. "Wellness as Virtue: Morality and the Pursuit of Health." *Culture, Medicine and Psychiatry* 18 (3): 385–401.

———. 2007. *The Medicalization of Society: On the Transformation of Human Conditions into Treatable Disorders*. Baltimore, MD: Johns Hopkins University Press.

Conrad, Peter, and Kristin K. Barker. 2010. "The Social Construction of Illness: Key Insights and Policy Implications." *Journal of Health and Social Behavior* 51 (Suppl.): S67–S79.

Conti, Allie. 2017. "South Florida's Most Infamous Butt Doctor Was Sentenced to Ten Years in Prison." *Vice*, March 28, 2017. https://www.vice.com/en_us/article/kbjpdw /south-floridas-most-infamous-butt-doctor-was-sentenced-to-ten-years-in-prison.

Cooper, Brittney. 2010. "A'n't I a Lady? Race Women, Michelle Obama, and the Ever-Expanding Democratic Imagination." *MELUS* 35 (4): 39–57.

Cooper, Charlotte. 2010. "Fat Studies: Mapping the Field." *Sociology Compass* 4 (12): 1020–1034.

Cooper, Wilbert L. 2015. "Why Smart Women Are Killing Themselves with Illegal Butt Injections." *Vice*, June 4, 2015. https://www.vice.com/en_us/article/jma8b7/why -women-are-getting-underground-butt-injections-456.

Correa, Sonia, and Rosalind Petchesky. 1994. "Reproductive and Sexual Rights: A Feminist Perspective." In *Population Policies Reconsidered: Health, Empowerment, and Rights*, ed. Gita Sen, Adrienne Germain, and Lincoln C. Chen. Boston, MA: Harvard University Press.

Courtenay, Will H. 2000. "Constructions of Masculinity and Their Influence on Men's Well-Being: A Theory of Gender and Health." *Social Science & Medicine* 50 (10): 1385–1401.

Crais, Clifton C., and Pamela Scully. 2009. *Sara Baartman and the Hottentot Venus: A Ghost Story and a Biography*. Princeton, NJ: Princeton University Press.

Crenshaw, Kimberlé. 1991. "Mapping the Margins: Intersectionality, Identity Politics, and Violence against Women of Color." *Stanford Law Review* 43 (6): 1241–1299.

Crocker, Lizzie. 2015. "Britain's Crazy Decision to Ban 'Beach Body' Ads." *The Daily Beast*, April 30, 2015. http://www.thedailybeast.com/articles/2015/04/30/britain-s-crazy -decision-to-ban-beach-body-ads.html.

Crocker, Lizzie, and Caitlin Dickson. 2012. "Illegal Butt Injections Are on the Rise and Women Are at Risk." *The Daily Beast*, October 13, 2012. https://www.thedailybeast .com/illegal-butt-injections-are-on-the-rise-and-women-are-at-risk.

Crowder, Kyle. 2000. "The Racial Context of White Mobility: An Individual-Level Assessment of the White Flight Hypothesis." *Social Science Research* 29 (2): 223–257.

Cryle, Peter, and Alison Moore. 2012. *Frigidity: An Intellectual History.* New York: Palgrave Macmillan.

Cunningham, Erin. 2014. "Our Photoshopping Disorder: The Truth in Advertising Bill Asks Congress to Regulate Deceptive Images." *The Daily Beast*, April 22, 2014. http://www.thedailybeast.com/articles/2014/04/22/our-photoshopping-disorder-the -truth-in-advertising-bill-asks-congress-to-regulate-deceptive-images.html.

Daar, Judith. 2017. *The New Eugenics: Selective Breeding in an Era of Reproductive Technologies.* New Haven, CT: Yale University Press.

Daley, Andrea, and Nick J. Mulé. 2014. "LGBTQs and the DSM-5: A Critical Queer Response." *Journal of Homosexuality* 61 (9): 1288–1312.

Daniels, Norman. 2000. "Normal Functioning and the Treatment-Enhancement Distinction." *Cambridge Quarterly of Healthcare Ethics* 9 (3): 309–322.

———. 2001. "Justice, Health, and Healthcare." *American Journal of Bioethics* 1 (2): 2–16.

———. 2007. *Just Health: Meeting Health Needs Fairly.* Cambridge, UK: Cambridge University Press.

David, Emmanuel. 2017. "Capital T Trans Visibility, Corporate Capitalism, and Commodity Culture." *TSQ: Transgender Studies Quarterly* 4 (1): 28–44.

Davis, Daniel. 2004. "Efficacy of Testosterone Transdermal System (TTS) for Treatment of HSDD in Surgically Menopausal Women on Concomitant Estrogen." Presented at the FDA Advisory Committee for Reproductive Health Drugs Meeting, Gaithersburg, MD, December 2.

Davis, Georgiann. 2015. *Contesting Intersex: The Dubious Diagnosis.* New York: New York University Press.

Davis, Georgiann, Jodie M. Dewey, and Erin L. Murphy. 2016. "Giving Sex: Deconstructing Intersex and Trans Medicalization Practices." *Gender & Society* 30 (3): 490–514.

Davis, Kathy. 1994. *Reshaping the Female Body: The Dilemma of Cosmetic Surgery.* New York: Routledge.

Davis, Lennard J. 1995. *Enforcing Normalcy: Disability, Deafness, and the Body.* London: Verso.

Daykin, Norma, and Jennie Naidoo. 1995. "Feminist Critiques of Health Promotion." In *The Sociology of Health Promotion: Critical Analyses of Consumption, Lifestyle and Risk*, ed. Robin Bunton, Sarah Nettleton, and Roger Burrows, 57–68. London: Routledge.

Derose, Kathryn Pitkin, Carole Roan Gresenz, and Jeanne S. Ringel. 2011. "Understanding Disparities in Health Care Access—and Reducing Them—through a Focus on Public Health." *Health Affairs* 30 (10): 1844–1851.

Derrida, Jacques. 1996. *The Gift of Death*. Chicago: University of Chicago Press.

———. 1999. *Adieu to Emmanuel Levinas*. Translated by Pascale-Anne Brault and Michael Naas. Stanford, CA: Stanford University Press.

———. 2006. *The Politics of Friendship*. Translated by George Collins. London: Verso.

"Detransition | Third Way Trans." n.d. Accessed April 20, 2017. https://thirdwaytrans .com/tag/detransition/.

Dewey, Caitlin. 2014. "Hate the Way Advertisers Photoshop Women's Bodies? So Does the Rep. Who Proposed This Anti-Photoshop Act." *Washington Post*, April 18, 2014. https://www.washingtonpost.com/news/arts-and-entertainment/wp/2014/04/18/hate -the-way-advertisers-photoshop-womens-bodies-so-does-the-rep-who-proposed -this-anti-photoshop-act/.

Dewey, Jodie M., and Melissa M. Gesbeck. 2017. "(Dys)Functional Diagnosing: Mental Health Diagnosis, Medicalization, and the Making of Transgender Patients." *Humanity & Society* 41 (1): 37–72.

Díaz, Rafael M., Andrea L. Heckert, and Jorge Sánchez. 2005. "Reasons for Stimulant Use among Latino Gay Men in San Francisco: A Comparison between Methamphetamine and Cocaine Users." *Journal of Urban Health* 82 (1): i71–i78.

Dickason, R. Myles, Vijai Chauhan, Astha Mor, Erin Ibler, Sarah Kuehnle, Daren Mahoney, Eric Armbrecht, and Preeti Dalawari. 2015. "Racial Differences in Opiate Administration for Pain Relief at an Academic Emergency Department." *Western Journal of Emergency Medicine* 16 (3): 372–380.

Donaghue, Ngaire, and Anne Clemitshaw. 2012. "'I'm Totally Smart and a Feminist . . . and yet I Want to Be a Waif': Exploring Ambivalence towards the Thin Ideal within the Fat Acceptance Movement." *Women's Studies International Forum* 35 (6): 415–425.

Downing, Lisa, Iain Morland, and Nikki Sullivan. 2014. *Fuckology: Critical Essays on John Money's Diagnostic Concepts*. Chicago: University of Chicago Press.

Dreger, Alice Domurat. 2009. *Hermaphrodites and the Medical Invention of Sex*. Boston, MA: Harvard University Press.

Drescher, Jack, Peggy Cohen-Kettenis, and Sam Winter. 2012. "Minding the Body: Situating Gender Identity Diagnoses in the ICD-11." *International Review of Psychiatry* 24 (6): 568–577.

Drew, Jennifer. 2003. "The Myth of Female Sexual Dysfunction and Its Medicalization." *Psychology, Evolution & Gender* 5 (2): 89–96.

Drew, Patricia. 2011. "'But Then I Learned . . .': Weight Loss Surgery Patients Negotiate Surgery Discourses." *Social Science & Medicine* 73 (8): 1230–1237.

Dreyfus, Tom. 2012. "The 'Half-Invention' of Gender Identity in International Human Rights Law: From Cedaw to the Yogyakarta Principles." *Australian Feminist Law Journal* 37 (December): 33–50.

Drum, Kevin. 2016. "A Very Brief Timeline of the Bathroom Wars." *Mother Jones*, May 14, 2016. http://www.motherjones.com/kevin-drum/2016/05/timeline-bathroom-wars/.

DTB. 2009. "Testosterone Patches for Female Sexual Dysfunction." *Drug and Therapeutics Bulletin* 47 (3): 30–34.

Duggan, Lisa. 2002. "The New Homonormativity: The Sexual Politics of Neoliberalism." In *Materializing Democracy: Toward a Revitalized Cultural Politics,* ed. Russ Castronovo and Dana D. Nelson, 175-194. Durham: Duke University Press.

Dussauge, Isabelle, and Anelis Kaiser. 2012. "Neuroscience and Sex/Gender." *Neuroethics*, 5 (3): 211-215.

Duster, Troy. 2006. "Lessons from History: Why Race and Ethnicity Have Played a Major Role in Biomedical Research." *Journal of Law, Medicine & Ethics* 34 (3): 487–496.

Edelman, Lee. 2004. *No Future: Queer Theory and the Death Drive*. Durham: Duke University Press.

Ehrenreich, Barbara, and Deirdre English. 2013. *For Her Own Good: Two Centuries of the Experts Advice to Women*. New York: Anchor.

Ekins, Richard. 2005. "Science, Politics and Clinical Intervention: Harry Benjamin, Transsexualism and the Problem of Heteronormativity." *Sexualities* 8 (3): 306–328.

England, Kim V. L. 1993. "Changing Suburbs, Changing Women: Geographic Perspectives on Suburban Women and Suburbanization." *Frontiers: A Journal of Women Studies* 14 (1): 24–43.

Erickson-Schroth, Laura. 2014. *Trans Bodies, Trans Selves: A Resource for the Transgender Community*. Oxford, UK: Oxford University Press.

Ernsberger, Paul. 2009. "Does Social Class Explain the Connection between Weight and Health." In *The Fat Studies Reader*, ed. Esther Rothblum and Sondra Solovay, 25–36. New York: NYU Press.

Escobar, Sam Escobar. 2016. "Woman with Cement in Her Face Gets Help from Plastic Surgeons." *Good Housekeeping*, May 12, 2016. http://www.goodhousekeeping.com/beauty/news/a38436/woman-with-cement-in-her-face-botched/.

Faith, Daniel P. 2016. "Biodiversity." In *The Stanford Encyclopedia of Philosophy*, ed. Edward N. Zalta. Metaphysics Research Lab, Stanford University. https://plato.stanford.edu/archives/sum2016/entries/biodiversity/.

Fallin-Bennett, Keisa. 2015. "Implicit Bias against Sexual Minorities in Medicine: Cycles of Professional Influence and the Role of the Hidden Curriculum." *Academic Medicine: Journal of the Association of American Medical Colleges* 90 (5): 549–552.

"A 'Fat Studies' Scholar No Longer Fits the Picture." 2006. *The Chronicle of Higher Education*. June 30, 2006. http://www.chronicle.com/article/A-Fat-Studies-Scholar-No/33887/?key=6TQovNhpONVPSS_S7KKKt8MWEEQYtvbpbPHBxaAxx2KlCVg1vgDXhQ9GCxoCQFfgb3VFNDZXN3lDaVROSXZzMHVsXo9zSVoyUjBSbzRGZm-J5TnlqSohvZo1EWQ.

Fausto-Sterling, Anne. 2005. "The Bare Bones of Sex: Part 1—Sex and Gender." *Signs: Journal of Women in Culture & Society* 30 (2): 1491–1527.

Featherstone, Mike. 2007. *Consumer Culture and Postmodernism*. Los Angeles: SAGE.

Ferguson, Roderick A. 2003. *Aberrations in Black: Toward a Queer of Color Critique*. Minneapolis: University of Minnesota Press.

Finney Rutten, Lila, Amy Lazarus Yaroch, Heather Patrick, Mary Story, Lila Finney Rutten, Amy Lazarus Yaroch, Heather Patrick, and Mary Story. 2012. "Obesity Prevention and National Food Security: A Food Systems Approach." *International Scholarly Research Notices* 2012 (November): e539764.

Fischer, Erin McKelle. 2015. "9 Body Positive Social Media Campaigns That Are Changing How We Perceive Beauty Both in and outside the Fashion World." *Bustle*, April 15, 2015. http://www.bustle.com/articles/75539-9-body-positive-social-media-campaigns-that-are-changing-how-we-perceive-beauty-both-in-and.

Fisher, Jill A. 2013. "Expanding the Frame of 'Voluntariness' in Informed Consent: Structural Coercion and the Power of Social and Economic Context." *Kennedy Institute of Ethics Journal* 23 (4): 355–379.

Fishman, Jennifer R. 2004. "Manufacturing Desire:" *Social Studies of Science* 34 (2): 187–218.

———. 2009. "The Biomedicalization of Sexual Dysfunction." In *Biomedicalization: Technoscience, Health, and Illness in the US*, ed. Adele E. Clarke, Laura Mamo, Jennifer Ruth Fosket, Jennifer R. Fishman, and Janet K. Shim, 289–306. Durham, NC: Duke University Press.

Fishman, Sara. 1998. "Life in the Fat Underground." *Radiance*, Winter 1998. http://www.radiancemagazine.com/issues/1998/winter_98/fat_underground.html.

Fletcher, Guy. 2016. *The Philosophy of Well-Being: An Introduction*. London: Routledge.

Flore, Jacinthe. 2013. "HSDD and Asexuality: A Question of Instruments." *Psychology and Sexuality* 4 (2): 152–166.

———. 2014. "Mismeasures of Asexual Desires." In *Asexualities: Feminist and Queer Perspectives*, ed. Karli June Cerankowski and Megan Milks, 17–34. New York: Routledge.

Food and Drug Administration (FDA). 2004. *Public Meeting on Intrinsa*. Gaithersburg, MD.

Food and Drug Administration (FDA). 2015. "Press Announcements—FDA Approves First Treatment for Sexual Desire Disorder." WebContent. August 18, 2015. http://www.fda.gov/NewsEvents/Newsroom/PressAnnouncements/ucm458734.htm.

Foucault, Michel. 1990. *The History of Sexuality: Vol. 1. An Introduction*. Translated by Robert Hurley. New York: Vintage Books, Random House.

———. 1994. *The Birth of the Clinic: An Archaeology of Medical Perception*. New York: Vintage.

Fowlkes, Diane L. 1997. "Moving from Feminist Identity Politics to Coalition Politics through a Feminist Materialist Standpoint of Intersubjectivity in Gloria Anzaldúa's Borderlands/La Frontera: The New Mestiza." *Hypatia* 12 (2): 105–124.

Freedman, Estelle B. 2013. *Redefining Rape*. Boston, MA: Harvard University Press.

Friedlander, Henry. 1997. *The Origins of Nazi Genocide: From Euthanasia to the Final Solution*. Chapel Hill: University of North Carolina Press.

Fullagar, Simone. 2009. "Negotiating the Neurochemical Self: Anti-Depressant Consumption in Women's Recovery from Depression." *Health:* 13 (4): 389–406.

Furet, Jean-Pierre, Ling-Chun Kong, Julien Tap, Christine Poitou, Arnaud Basdevant, Jean-Luc Bouillot, Denis Mariat, et al. 2010. "Differential Adaptation of Human Gut Microbiota to Bariatric Surgery–Induced Weight Loss." *Diabetes* 59 (12): 3049–3057.

Gabriel, Joseph M., and Daniel S. Goldberg. 2014. "Big Pharma and the Problem of Disease Inflation." *International Journal of Health Services* 44 (2): 307–322.

Gaesser, Glenn. 2009. "Is 'Permanent Weight Loss' an Oxymoron? The Statistics on Weight Loss and the National Weight Control Registry." In *The Fat Studies Reader*, ed. Esther Rothblum and Sondra Solovay, 37–40. New York: NYU Press.

Gammell, Deanna J., and Janet M. Stoppard. 1999. "Women's Experiences of Treatment of Depression: Medicalization or Empowerment?" *Canadian Psychology/Psychologie Canadienne* 40 (2): 112–128.

Garland Thomson, Rosemarie. 1997. *Extraordinary Bodies: Figuring Physical Disability in American Culture and Literature*. New York: Columbia University Press.

Garland-Thomson, Rosemarie 2012. "The Case for Conserving Disability." *Journal of Bioethical Inquiry* 9 (3): 339–355.
———. 2017. "Eugenic World Building and Disability: The Strange World of Kazuo Ishiguro's Never Let Me Go." *Journal of Medical Humanities* 38 (2): 133–145.
Gavey, Nicola. 2005. *Just Sex? The Cultural Scaffolding of Rape.* New York: Routledge.
Gehi, Pooja S., and Gabriel Arkles. 2007. "Unraveling Injustice: Race and Class Impact of Medicaid Exclusions of Transition-Related Health Care for Transgender People." *Sexuality Research & Social Policy* 4 (4): 7.
"Getting Electrolysis Covered." n.d. Susan's Place Transgender Resources. Accessed April 18, 2017. https://www.susans.org/forums/index.php?topic=185364.0.
Gillespie, Rosemary. 1997. "Women, the Body and Brand Extension in Medicine." *Women & Health* 24 (4): 69–85.
Gill-Peterson, Julian. 2014. "The Technical Capacities of the Body: Assembling Race, Technology, and Transgender." *TSQ: Transgender Studies Quarterly* 1 (3): 402–418.
Gilman, Sander L. 1985. "Black Bodies, White Bodies: Toward an Iconography of Female Sexuality in Late Nineteenth-Century Art, Medicine, and Literature." *Critical Inquiry* 12 (1): 204–242.
Giordano, Simona. 2012. "Sliding Doors: Should Treatment of Gender Identity Disorder and Other Body Modifications Be Privately Funded?" *Medicine, Health Care and Philosophy* 15 (1): 31–40.
Giovanelli, Dina, and Natalie M. Peluso. 2006. "Feederism: A New Sexual Pleasure and Subculture." In *Handbook of New Sexuality Studies,* ed. Steven Seidman, Nancy Fischer, and Chet Meeks, 309–313. London: Routledge.
Gloy, Viktoria L., Matthias Briel, Deepak L. Bhatt, Sangeeta R. Kashyap, Philip R. Schauer, Geltrude Mingrone, Heiner C. Bucher, and Alain J. Nordmann. 2013. "Bariatric Surgery versus Non-Surgical Treatment for Obesity: A Systematic Review and Meta-Analysis of Randomised Controlled Trials." *BMJ* 347 (October): f5934.
Goldstein, Irwin, Tom F. Lue, Harin Padma-Nathan, Raymond C. Rosen, William D. Steers, and Pierre A. Wicker. 1998. "Oral Sildenafil in the Treatment of Erectile Dysfunction." *New England Journal of Medicine* 338 (20): 1397–1404.
Gordon-Larsen, Penny, Melissa C. Nelson, Phil Page, and Barry M. Popkin. 2006. "Inequality in the Built Environment Underlies Key Health Disparities in Physical Activity and Obesity." *Pediatrics* 117 (2): 417–424.
Grandin, Temple. n.d. "Evaluating the Effects of Medication on People with Autism." Autism Support Network. Accessed May 12, 2017. http://www.autismsupportnetwork.com/news/evaluating-effects-medication-autism-2292833.
Grewal, Inderpal. 1999. "'Women's Rights as Human Rights': Feminist Practices, Global Feminism, and Human Rights Regimes in Transnationality." *Citizenship Studies* 3 (3): 337–354.
Grey, Stephanie Houston. 2016. "Contesting the Fit Citizen: Michelle Obama and the Body Politics of *The Biggest Loser.*" *Journal of Popular Culture* 49 (3): 564–581.
Groneman, Carol. 2001. *Nymphomania: A History.* New York: W. W. Norton.
Grosz, Elizabeth. 1990. "A Note on Essentialism and Difference." In *Feminist Knowledge: Critique and Construct,* ed. Sneja Gunew, 332–344. London: Routledge.
Guay, A. 2005. "Commentary on Androgen Deficiency in Women and the FDA Advisory Board's Recent Decision to Request More Safety Data." *International Journal of Impotence Research* 17 (4): 375–376.

Guerrero, J. David. 2010. "On a Naturalist Theory of Health: A Critique." *Studies in History and Philosophy of Biological and Biomedical Sciences* 41 (3): 272–278.

Gunson, Jessica Shipman. 2010. "'More Natural but Less Normal': Reconsidering Medicalisation and Agency through Women's Accounts of Menstrual Suppression." *Social Science & Medicine* 71 (7): 1324–1331.

Gupta, Kristina. 2012. "Protecting Sexual Diversity: Rethinking the Use of Neurotechnological Interventions to Alter Sexuality." *American Journal of Bioethics Neuroscience* 3 (3): 24–28.

———. 2013a. "Compulsory Sexuality and Its Discontents: The Challenge of Asexualities." PhD diss., Emory University.

———. 2013b. "Happy Asexual Meets DSM." *SocialText Online (Periscope)*. DSM-CRIP (October). https://socialtextjournal.org/periscope_article/happy-asexual-meets-dsm/.

———. 2014. "Asexuality and Disability: Mutual Negation in Adams v. Rice and New Directions for Coalition Building." In *Asexualities: Feminist and Queer Perspectives*, ed. Karli June Cerankowski and Megan Milks. New York: Routledge.

———. 2015a. "Compulsory Sexuality: Evaluating an Emerging Concept." *Signs: Journal of Women in Culture & Society* 41 (1): 131–154.

———. 2015b. "What Does Asexuality Teach Us about Sexual Disinterest? Recommendations for Health Professionals Based on a Qualitative Study with Asexually Identified People." *Journal of Sex & Marital Therapy* 43 (1): 1–14.

———. 2017. "'And Now I'm Just Different, but There's Nothing Actually Wrong with Me': Asexual Marginalization and Resistance." *Journal of Homosexuality* 64 (8): 991–1013.

Gupta, Kristina, and Sara M. Freeman. 2013. "Preimplantation Genetic Diagnosis for Intersex Conditions: Beyond Parental Decision Making." *American Journal of Bioethics* 13 (10): 49–51.

Guthman, Julie. 2011. *Weighing In: Obesity, Food Justice, and the Limits of Capitalism.* Berkeley: University of California Press.

Halkitis, Perry N., and Kelly A. Green. 2007. "Sildenafil (Viagra) and Club Drug Use in Gay and Bisexual Men: The Role of Drug Combinations and Context." *American Journal of Men's Health* 1 (2): 139–147.

Hall, Kim Q. 2002. "Feminism, Disability, and Embodiment." *NWSA Journal* 14 (3): vii–xiii.

———. 2015. "Toward a Queer Crip Feminist Politics of Food." *PhiloSOPHIA* 4 (2): 177–196.

Hancock, Ange-Marie. 2016. *Intersectionality: An Intellectual History.* Oxford, UK: Oxford University Press.

Haraway, Donna. 1988. "Situated Knowledges: The Science Question in Feminism and the Privilege of Partial Perspective." *Feminist Studies* 14 (3): 575–599.

———. 1991a. *Simians, Cyborgs, and Women: The Reinvention of Nature.* New York: Routledge.

———. 1991b. "A Cyborg Manifesto: Science, Technology, and Socialist-Feminism in the Late Twentieth Century." In *Simians, Cyborgs and Women: The Reinvention of Nature*, 149–181. New York: Routledge.

———. 1997. *Modest_Witness@Second_Millennium.FemaleMan©_Meets_ OncoMouse: Feminism and Technoscience.* New York: Routledge.

———. 2003. *The Companion Species Manifesto: Dogs, People, and Significant Otherness.* Edited by Matthew Begelke. Chicago: Prickly Paradigm Press.

Harding, Sandra. 1986. *The Science Question in Feminism*. Ithaca, NY: Cornell University Press.

———, ed. 2003. *The Feminist Standpoint Theory Reader: Intellectual and Political Controversies*. New York: Routledge.

Hartley, Heather. 2006. "The 'Pinking' of Viagra Culture: Drug Industry Efforts to Create and Repackage Sex Drugs for Women." *Sexualities* 9 (3): 363–378.

Hartman, Saidiya V. 1997. *Scenes of Subjection: Terror, Slavery, and Self-Making in Nineteenth-Century America*. New York: Oxford University Press.

Hausman, Bernice L. 1995. *Changing Sex: Transsexualism, Technology, and the Idea of Gender*. Durham, NC: Duke University Press Books.

"Healthcare." n.d. National Center for Transgender Equality. Accessed April 18, 2017. http://www.transequality.org/know-your-rights/healthcare.

Healy, David. 2004. *Let Them Eat Prozac: The Unhealthy Relationship between the Pharmaceutical Industry and Depression*. New York: New York University Press.

Heather, Stephenson, and Kiki Zeldes. 2008. "'Write a Chapter and Change the World': How the Boston Women's Health Book Collective Transformed Women's Health Then—and Now." *American Journal of Public Health* 98 (10): 1741–1745.

Heiman, J. R., D. R. Talley, J. L. Bailen, T. A. Oskin, S. J. Rosenberg, C. R. Pace, D. L. Creanga, and T. Bavendam. 2007. "Sexual Function and Satisfaction in Heterosexual Couples When Men Are Administered Sildenafil Citrate (Viagra) for Erectile Dysfunction: A Multicentre, Randomised, Double-Blind, Placebo-Controlled Trial." *BJOG: An International Journal of Obstetrics and Gynaecology* 114 (4): 437–447.

Heins, Janet Kaye, Alan Heins, Marianthe Grammas, Melissa Costello, Kun Huang, and Satya Mishra. 2006. "Disparities in Analgesia and Opioid Prescribing Practices for Patients with Musculoskeletal Pain in the Emergency Department." *Journal of Emergency Nursing* 32 (3): 219–224.

Heldman, Breanne L. 2009. "Chaz Bono: Gender Is between Your Ears, Not Legs." *E! Online*, November 19, 2009. http://www.eonline.com/news/154521/chaz-bono-gender-is-between-your-ears-not-legs.

Herndon, April. 2002. "Disparate but Disabled: Fat Embodiment and Disability Studies." *NWSA Journal* 14 (3): 120–137.

Heyes, Cressida J. 2006. "Foucault Goes to Weight Watchers." *Hypatia* 21 (2): 126–149.

———. 2007. *Self-Transformations: Foucault, Ethics, and Normalized Bodies*. Oxford, UK: Oxford University Press.

Hiatt, William R., Abraham Thomas, and Allison B. Goldfine. 2012. "What Cost Weight Loss?" *Circulation* 125 (9): 1171–1177.

Hinderliter, Andrew. 2009. "Hypoactive Sexual Desire Disorder and the Asexual Community: A History." *Asexual Explorations Blog* (blog). March 28, 2009. http://asexystuff.blogspot.com/2009/03/hypoactive-sexual-desire-disorder-and.html.

Hines, Sally. 2009. "A Pathway to Diversity? Human Rights, Citizenship and the Politics of Transgender." *Contemporary Politics* 15 (1): 87–102.

Hite, Shere. 2011. *The Hite Report: A Nationwide Study of Female Sexuality*. New York: Seven Stories Press.

Hiza, Hazel A. B., Kellie O. Casavale, Patricia M. Guenther, and Carole A. Davis. 2013. "Diet Quality of Americans Differs by Age, Sex, Race/Ethnicity, Income, and Education Level." *Journal of the Academy of Nutrition and Dietetics* 113 (2): 297–306.

Hochschild, Arlie, and Anne Machung. 2012. *The Second Shift: Working Families and the Revolution at Home*. Rev. ed. New York: Penguin Books.

Hollenberg, Daniel, and Linda Muzzin. 2010. "Epistemological Challenges to Integrative Medicine: An Anti-Colonial Perspective on the Combination of Complementary/Alternative Medicine with Biomedicine." *Health Sociology Review* 19 (1): 34–56.

Huang, Alison J., Leslee L. Subak, David H. Thom, Stephen K. Van Den Eeden, Arona I. Ragins, Miriam Kuppermann, Hui Shen, and Jeanette S. Brown. 2009. "Sexual Function and Aging in Racially and Ethnically Diverse Women." *Journal of the American Geriatrics Society* 57 (8): 1362–1368.

Hubbard, Ruth. 2013. "Abortion and Disability: Who Should and Who Should Not Inhabit the World." In *The Disability Studies Reader*, ed. Lennard J. Davis, 4th ed., 74–86. New York: Routledge.

Hurley, Elisa A. 2010. "Pharmacotherapy to Blunt Memories of Sexual Violence: What's a Feminist to Think?" *Hypatia* 25 (3): 527–552.

"ICATH." n.d. ICATH. Accessed April 6, 2017. https://icath.info/.

International Network for Trans Depathologization. n.d. "Manifesto." Stop Trans Pathologization. Accessed April 24, 2017. http://www.stp2012.info/old/en/manifesto.

Irvine, Janice M. 2005. *Disorders of Desire: Sexuality and Gender in Modern American Sexology*. Rev. and expanded. Philadelphia, PA: Temple University Press.

Irving, Dan. 2008. "Normalized Transgressions: Legitimizing the Transsexual Body as Productive." *Radical History Review* 2008 (100): 38–59.

"Is There Any Way to Get Laser or Electrolysis Covered under Insurance?" n.d. Reddit Asktransgender. Accessed April 18, 2017. https://www.reddit.com/r/asktransgender/comments/2m2r42/is_there_any_way_to_get_laser_or_electrolysis/.

Jackson, Alyssa. n.d. "The High Cost of Being Transgender." CNN. Accessed April 18, 2017. http://www.cnn.com/2015/07/31/health/transgender-costs-irpt/index.html.

Jacobs, Julia. 2018. "Trump Administration Rolls Back Obama-Era Rules for School Lunches." *New York Times*, December 9, 2018. https://www.nytimes.com/2018/12/08/us/trump-school-lunch-usda.html.

Jarrin, Alvaro E. 2012. "The Rise of the Cosmetic Nation: Plastic Governmentality and Hybrid Medical Practices in Brazil." *Medical Anthropology* 31 (3): 213–228.

Jeffreys, Sheila. 2014. *Gender Hurts: A Feminist Analysis of the Politics of Transgenderism*. Abingdon, UK: Routledge.

Jneid, Hani, Gregg C. Fonarow, Christopher P. Cannon, Adrian F. Hernandez, Igor F. Palacios, Andrew O. Maree, Quinn Wells, et al. 2008. "Sex Differences in Medical Care and Early Death After Acute Myocardial Infarction." *Circulation* 118 (25): 2803–2810.

Joffe, Hylton V., Christina Chang, Catherine Sewell, Olivia Easley, Christine Nguyen, Somya Dunn, Kimberly Lehrfeld, et al. 2016. "FDA Approval of Flibanserin—Treating Hypoactive Sexual Desire Disorder." *New England Journal of Medicine* 374 (2): 101–104.

Johnson, Austin H. 2015. "Normative Accountability: How the Medical Model Influences Transgender Identities and Experiences." *Sociology Compass* 9 (9): 803–813.

———. 2016. "Transnormativity: A New Concept and Its Validation through Documentary Film about Transgender Men." *Sociological Inquiry* 86 (4): 465–491.

Jonassen, Jennifer. 2011. "Weight Stigma: Breaking It Down with Advocate and Activist Marilyn Wann." *Adios Barbie* (blog). September 27, 2011. http://www.adiosbarbie.com/2011/09/weight-stigma-breaking-it-down-with-advocate-and-activist-marilyn-wann/.

Jutel, Annemarie. 2001. "Does Size Really Matter? Weight and Values in Public Health." *Perspectives in Biology and Medicine* 44 (2): 283–296.

———. 2005. "Weighing Health: The Moral Burden of Obesity." *Social Semiotics* 15 (2): 113–125.

———. 2010. "Framing Disease: The Example of Female Hypoactive Sexual Desire Disorder." *Social Science & Medicine* 70 (7): 1084–1090.

Kaestner, Robert. 2009. "Obesity: Causes, Consequences and Public Solutions." The *Illinois Report 2009*. Urbana: The Institute of Government and Public Affairs at the University of Illinois.

Kafer, Alison. 2013. *Feminist, Queer, Crip*. Bloomington: Indiana University Press.

Karkazis, Katrina. 2008. *Fixing Sex: Intersex, Medical Authority, and Lived Experience*. Durham, NC: Duke University Press.

Karmali, Shahzeer. 2013. "The Impact of Bariatric Surgery on Psychological Health." *Journal of Obesity* 2013: 837989.

Keller, Evelyn Fox. 1992. *Secrets of Life, Secrets of Death: Essays on Language, Gender and Science*. New York: Routledge.

Kerner, Ian. 2004. *She Comes First: The Thinking Man's Guide to Pleasuring a Woman*. New York: HarperCollins.

Kessler, Suzanne J. 1998. *Lessons from the Intersexed*. Rutgers, NJ: Rutgers University Press.

Khan, Huma. 2010. "Michelle Obama on Obesity: Too Personal?" *ABC News*, February 5, 2010. https://abcnews.go.com/Politics/Health/michelle-obama-obesity-comments-bring ing-malia-sasha-wrong/story?id=9751138.

Khera, Rohan, Mohammad Hassan Murad, Apoorva K. Chandar, Parambir S. Dulai, Zhen Wang, Larry J. Prokop, Rohit Loomba, Michael Camilleri, and Siddharth Singh. 2016. "Association of Pharmacological Treatments for Obesity with Weight Loss and Adverse Events: A Systematic Review and Meta-Analysis." *JAMA* 315 (22): 2424–2434.

Kilbourne, Jean. 2004. "'The More You Subtract, the More You Add': Cutting Girls Down to Size." In *Psychology and Consumer Culture: The Struggle for a Good Life in a Materialistic World*, ed. T. Kasser and A. D. Kanner, 251–270. Washington, D.C.: American Psychological Association.

Kim, Eunjung. 2010. "How Much Sex Is Healthy? The Pleasures of Asexuality." In *Against Health: How Health Became the New Morality*, ed. Jonathan Metzl and Anna Kirkland, 157–169. New York: New York University Press.

———. 2011. "Asexuality in Disability Narratives." *Sexualities* 14 (4): 479–493.

Kim, Scott Y. H. 2011. "The Ethics of Informed Consent in Alzheimer Disease Research." *Nature Reviews Neurology* 7 (7): 410–414.

King, Samantha. 2004. "Pink Ribbons Inc: Breast Cancer Activism and the Politics of Philanthropy." *International Journal of Qualitative Studies in Education* 17 (4): 473–492.

Kingma, Elselijn. 2007. "What Is It to Be Healthy?" *Analysis* 67 (294): 128–133.

———. 2014. "Naturalism about Health and Disease: Adding Nuance for Progress." *Journal of Medicine and Philosophy: A Forum for Bioethics and Philosophy of Medicine* 39 (6): 590–608.

Kingsberg, Sheryl A. 2005. "The Testosterone Patch for Women." *International Journal of Impotence Research* 17 (5): 465–466.

Kirby, Vicki. 1991. "Corporeal Habits: Addressing Essentialism Differently." *Hypatia* 6 (3): 4–24.

————. 1997. *Telling Flesh: The Substance of the Corporeal*. New York: Routledge.

Kirkland, Anna. 2011. "The Environmental Account of Obesity: A Case for Feminist Skepticism." *Signs* 36 (2): 463–485.

Klawiter, Maren. 2008. *The Biopolitics of Breast Cancer: Changing Cultures of Disease and Activism*. Minneapolis: University of Minnesota Press.

Kleege, Georgina. 1999. *Sight Unseen*. New Haven, CT: Yale University Press.

Klesse, Christian. 2007. "Racialising the Politics of Transgression: Body Modification in Queer Culture." *Social Semiotics* 17 (3): 275–292.

Kline, Wendy. 2001. *Building a Better Race: Gender, Sexuality, and Eugenics from the Turn of the Century to the Baby Boom*. Berkeley: University of California Press.

Kluge, Eike-Henner W. 2005. "Competence, Capacity, and Informed Consent: Beyond the Cognitive-Competence Model." *Canadian Journal on Aging / La Revue Canadienne Du Vieillissement* 24 (3): 295–304.

Kollman, Kelly, and Matthew Waites. 2009. "The Global Politics of Lesbian, Gay, Bisexual and Transgender Human Rights: An Introduction." *Contemporary Politics* 15 (1): 1–17.

Kong, Ling-Chun, Julien Tap, Judith Aron-Wisnewsky, Veronique Pelloux, Arnaud Basdevant, Jean-Luc Bouillot, Jean-Daniel Zucker, Joël Doré, and Karine Clément. 2013. "Gut Microbiota after Gastric Bypass in Human Obesity: Increased Richness and Associations of Bacterial Genera with Adipose Tissue Genes." *American Journal of Clinical Nutrition* 98 (1): 16–24.

Koven, Suzanne. 2013. "Diet Drugs Work: Why Won't Doctors Prescribe Them?" *New Yorker*, December 4, 2013. http://www.newyorker.com/tech/elements/diet-drugs-work-why-wont-doctors-prescribe-them.

Krag, Erik. 2014. "Health as Normal Function: A Weak Link in Daniels's Theory of Just Health Distribution." *Bioethics* 28 (8): 427–435.

Kraus, Cynthia. 2015. "Classifying Intersex in DSM-5: Critical Reflections on Gender Dysphoria." *Archives of Sexual Behavior* 44 (5): 1147–1163.

Kulick, Don. 1998. *Travesti: Sex, Gender, and Culture among Brazilian Transgendered Prostitutes*. Chicago: University of Chicago Press.

Kumanyika, Shiriki K., Eva Obarzanek, Nicolas Stettler, Ronny Bell, Alison E. Field, Stephen P. Fortmann, Barry A. Franklin, et al. 2008. "Population-Based Prevention of Obesity." *Circulation* 118 (4): 428–464.

Kumari, Veena, and Peggy Postma. 2005. "Nicotine Use in Schizophrenia: The Self Medication Hypotheses." *Neuroscience & Biobehavioral Reviews* 29 (6): 1021–1034.

Kurz, Demie. 1987. "Emergency Department Responses to Battered Women: Resistance to Medicalization." *Social Problems* 34 (1): 69–81.

Laan, Ellen, Rik H. W. van Lunsen, Walter Everaerd, Alan Riley, Elizabeth Scott, and Mitradev Boolell. 2002. "The Enhancement of Vaginal Vasocongestion by Sildenafil in Healthy Premenopausal Women." *Journal of Women's Health & Gender-Based Medicine* 11 (4): 357–365.

Laine, Christine, and Barbara J. Turner. 2004. "Unequal Pay for Equal Work: The Gender Gap in Academic Medicine." *Annals of Internal Medicine; Philadelphia* 141 (3): 238–240.

Langer, Susan J., and James I. Martin. 2004. "How Dresses Can Make You Mentally Ill: Examining Gender Identity Disorder in Children." *Child and Adolescent Social Work Journal* 21 (1): 5–23.

Laumann, Edward O., Anthony Paik, and Raymond C. Rosen. 1999. "Sexual Dysfunction in the United States: Prevalence and Predictors." *JAMA* 281 (6): 537–544.

Lavis, Victoria, Christine Horrocks, Nancy Kelly, and Val Barker. 2005. "Domestic Violence and Health Care: Opening Pandora's Box—Challenges and Dilemmas." *Feminism & Psychology* 15 (4): 441–460.

LeBesco, Kathleen. 2004. *Revolting Bodies? The Struggle to Redefine Fat Identity.* Boston: University of Massachusetts Press.

———. 2009a. "Quest for a Cause: The Fat Gene, the Gay Gene, and the New Eugenics." In *The Fat Studies Reader*, ed. Esther Rothblum and Sondra Solovay, 65–74. New York: NYU Press.

———. 2009b. "Weight Management, Good Health and the Will to Normality." In *Critical Feminist Approaches to Eating Dis/Orders*, ed. Helen Malson and Maree Burns, 146–155. New York: Routledge.

———. 2011. "Neoliberalism, Public Health, and the Moral Perils of Fatness." *Critical Public Health* 21 (2): 153–164.

———. 2015. "Fat." In *Keywords for Disability Studies*, ed. Rachel Adams, Benjamin Reiss, and David Serlin, 84. New York: New York University Press.

———. 2016. "On Fatness and Fluidity: A Meditation." In *Queering Fat Embodiment*, ed. Cat Pausé, Samantha Murray, and Jackie Wykes, 64–75. New York: Routledge.

Leblanc, Vicky, Véronique Provencher, Catherine Bégin, Louise Corneau, Angelo Tremblay, and Simone Lemieux. 2012. "Impact of a Health-At-Every-Size Intervention on Changes in Dietary Intakes and Eating Patterns in Premenopausal Overweight Women: Results of a Randomized Trial." *Clinical Nutrition* 31 (4): 481–488.

Leigh, Danielle, and Susan Hess Logeais. 2014. "Can Plastic Surgery Be Liberating?" *New Internationalist*, July 2014. https://newint.org/sections/argument/2014/07/01/can-plastic-surgery-be-liberating/.

Lenzer, Jeanne. 2010. "Boehringer Ingelheim Withdraws Libido Drug for Women." *BMJ* 341: c5701.

Levine, Philippa. 1994. "Venereal Disease, Prostitution, and the Politics of Empire: The Case of British India." *Journal of the History of Sexuality* 4 (4): 579–602.

Lewis, Linwood J. 2004. "Examining Sexual Health Discourses in a Racial/Ethnic Context." *Archives of Sexual Behavior* 33 (3): 223–234.

Little, Margaret Olivia. 1998. "Cosmetic Surgery, Suspect Norms, and the Ethics of Complicity." In *Enhancing Human Traits: Ethical and Social Implications*, ed. Erik Parens, 162–176. Washington, D.C.: Georgetown University Press.

Lloyd, Moya. 2007. "(Women's) Human Rights: Paradoxes and Possibilities." *Review of International Studies* 33 (1): 91–103.

Lock, Margaret M. 1994. *Encounters with Aging: Mythologies of Menopause in Japan and North America.* Berkeley: University of California Press.

Loe, Meika. 2001. "Fixing Broken Masculinity: Viagra as a Technology for the Production of Gender and Sexuality." *Sexuality and Culture* 5 (3): 97–125.

Lohr, Kathy. n.d. "Controversy Swirls Around Harsh Anti-Obesity Ads." *NPR.org*. Accessed January 11, 2017. http://www.npr.org/2012/01/09/144799538/controversy-swirls-around-harsh-anti-obesity-ads.

Lombardo, Paul A. 2010. *Three Generations, No Imbeciles: Eugenics, the Supreme Court, and Buck v. Bell.* Baltimore: Johns Hopkins University Press.

———. 2015. "How to Escape the Doctor's Dilemma? De-Medicalize Reproductive Technologies." *Journal of Law, Medicine & Ethics* 43 (2): 326–329.

Lomelino, Pamela J. 2015. *Community, Autonomy and Informed Consent: Revisiting the Philosophical Foundation for Informed Consent in International Research.* Newcastle, UK: Cambridge Scholars Publishing.

Longhurst, Robyn. 2012. "Becoming Smaller: Autobiographical Spaces of Weight Loss." *Antipode* 44 (3): 871–888.

Longino, Helen E. 1990. *Science as Social Knowledge.* Princeton, NJ: Princeton University Press.

Lopez, Russ. 2004. "Urban Sprawl and Risk for Being Overweight or Obese." *American Journal of Public Health* 94 (9): 1574–1579.

Lopez, Russell P., and H. Patricia Hynes. 2006. "Obesity, Physical Activity, and the Urban Environment: Public Health Research Needs." *Environmental Health* 5: 25.

Lorber, Judith. 1994. *Paradoxes of Gender.* New Haven, CT: Yale University Press.

Lorber, Judith, and Lisa Jean Moore. 2002. *Gender and the Social Construction of Illness.* Lanham, MD: Altamira.

Lorde, Audre. 1980. *The Cancer Journals.* San Francisco: Aunt Lute Books.

———. 1984. *Sister Outsider: Essays and Speeches.* Berkeley, CA: Crossing Press.

———. 2017. *A Burst of Light: And Other Essays.* Mineola, NY: Ixia Press.

Lucas, Johna D. 2004. "Phase III Surgical Menopause Efficacy Overview." Presented at the FDA Advisory Committee for Reproductive Health Drugs Meeting, Gaithersburg, MD, December 2.

Lucas, Liza. 2015. "Black Market Butt Injections: Dangerous and Deadly." *CNN*, June 24, 2015. http://www.cnn.com/2015/06/24/health/deadly-butt-injections/index.html.

Luckett, Sharrell D. 2014. "YoungGiftedandFat: Performing Transweight Identities." *Journal of American Drama and Theatre* 26 (2): 1–13.

Lupton, Deborah. 2012. "A Sociological Critique of the Health at Every Size Movement." *This Sociological Life* (blog). September 24, 2012. https://simplysociology.wordpress .com/2012/09/24/a-sociological-critique-of-the-health-at-every-size-movement/.

Lyons, Pat. 2009. "Prescription for Harm: Diet Industry Influence, Public Health Policy, and the 'Obesity Epidemic.'" In *The Fat Studies Reader*, ed. Esther Rothblum and Sondra Solovay, 75–87. New York: NYU Press.

MacDougall, Robert. 2006. "Remaking the Real Man: Erectile Dysfunction Palliatives and the Social Re-Construction of the Male Heterosexual Life Cycle." *Sexuality and Culture* 10 (3): 59–90.

MacKay, Jenna M., and Alexandra Rutherford. 2012. "Feminist Women's Accounts of Depression." *Affilia* 27 (2): 180–189.

Maclean, Alasdair. 2013. *Autonomy, Informed Consent and Medical Law: A Relational Challenge.* Reprint ed. Cambridge, UK: Cambridge University Press.

Macsta, Brandon. 2010. "An Open Letter to First Lady Michelle Obama." November 23, 2010. https://dailycaller.com/2010/11/23/open-letter-to-first-lady-michelle-obama/.

Magubane, Zine. 2001. "Which Bodies Matter? Feminism, Poststructuralism, Race, and the Curious Theoretical Odyssey of the 'Hottentot Venus.'" *Gender & Society* 15 (6): 816–834.

Mahalik, James R., Shaun M. Burns, and Matthew Syzdek. 2007. "Masculinity and Perceived Normative Health Behaviors as Predictors of Men's Health Behaviors." *Social Science & Medicine* 64 (11): 2201–2209.

Maines, Rachel P. 2001. *The Technology of Orgasm: "Hysteria," the Vibrator, and Women's Sexual Satisfaction*. Baltimore, MD: Johns Hopkins University Press.

Mairs, Nancy. 1997. *Waist-High in the World: A Life among the Nondisabled*. New ed. Boston: Beacon.

Mamo, Laura, and Jennifer Ruth Fosket. 2009. "Scripting the Body: Pharmaceuticals and the (Re)Making of Menstruation." *Signs: Journal of Women in Culture and Society* 34 (4): 925–949.

Mancini, E. 2010. *Magnus Hirschfeld and the Quest for Sexual Freedom: A History of the First International Sexual Freedom Movement*. New York: Palgrave MacMillan.

Manson, Neil C., and Onora O'Neill. 2007. *Rethinking Informed Consent in Bioethics*. Cambridge, UK: Cambridge University Press.

Marcum, James A. 2008. *An Introductory Philosophy of Medicine: Humanizing Modern Medicine*. New York: Springer.

Marshall, Barbara L. 2006. "The New Virility: Viagra, Male Aging and Sexual Function." *Sexualities* 9 (3): 345–362.

Marshall, Barbara L., and Stephen Katz. 2013. "From Androgyny to Androgens: Resexing the Aging Body." In *Age Matters: Realigning Feminist Thinking*, ed. Toni M. Calasanti and Kathleen F. Slevin. New York: Routledge.

Martin, Emily. 2001. *The Woman in the Body: A Cultural Analysis of Reproduction*. Boston: Beacon.

Martin, Matthew, Alec Beekley, Randy Kjorstad, and James Sebesta. 2010. "Socioeconomic Disparities in Eligibility and Access to Bariatric Surgery: A National Population-Based Analysis." *Surgery for Obesity and Related Diseases* 6 (1): 8–15.

Mayer, Jane. 2016. *Dark Money: The Hidden History of the Billionaires behind the Rise of the Radical Right*. New York: Doubleday.

Mayor, Susan. 2004. "Pfizer Will Not Apply for a Licence for Sildenafil for Women." *BMJ: British Medical Journal* 328 (7439): 542.

McAfee, Noëlle, and R. Claire Snyder. 2007. "Feminist Engagements in Democratic Theory." *Hypatia* 22 (4): vii–x.

McAllister, Heather. 2009. "Embodying Fat Liberation." In *The Fat Studies Reader*, ed. Esther Rothblum and Sondra Solovay, 305–311. New York: New York University Press.

McCall, Leslie. 2005. "The Complexity of Intersectionality." *Signs* 30 (3): 1771–1800.

McCune, Jeffrey Q. 2014. *Sexual Discretion: Black Masculinity and the Politics of Passing*. Chicago: University of Chicago Press.

McLaren, Angus. 2007. *Impotence: A Cultural History*. Chicago: University of Chicago Press.

McRuer, Robert. 2006. *Crip Theory: Cultural Signs of Queerness and Disability*. New York: NYU Press.

McShane, Thomas O., Paul D. Hirsch, Tran Chi Trung, Alexander N. Songorwa, Ann Kinzig, Bruno Monteferri, David Mutekanga, et al. 2011. "Hard Choices: Making Trade-Offs between Biodiversity Conservation and Human Well-Being." *Biological Conservation* 144 (3): 966–972.

Medical Board of California. 2007. "Consumer Corner: Medical Spas—What You Need to Know." *Medical Board of California Newsletter* 100 (January): 10.

"Medicare." n.d. National Center for Transgender Equality. Accessed April 6, 2017. http://www.transequality.org/know-your-rights/medicare.

Meleo-Erwin, Zoë C. 2011. "'A Beautiful Show of Strength': Weight Loss and the Fat Activist Self." *Health: An Interdisciplinary Journal for the Social Study of Health, Illness and Medicine* 15 (2): 188–205.

Mettler, Katie. 2017. "Fake Florida Doctor Who 'Enhanced' Buttocks with Cement, Caulking Gets 10 Years for Manslaughter." *Washington Post*, March 28, 2017. https://www.washingtonpost.com/news/morning-mix/wp/2017/03/28/woman-who-enhanced-butts-with-glue-and-cement-gets-10-years-for-manslaughter/?tid=pm_pop&utm_term=.5dfd658fc385.

Mettler, Katie, and *Washington Post*. 2017. "Florida's 'Toxic Tush' Fake Booty Enhancement Plastic Surgeon Gets 10 Years for Manslaughter." *Houston Chronicle*, March 28, 2017. http://www.chron.com/national/article/Florida-s-Toxic-Tush-fake-booty-enhancement-11033079.php.

Metzl, Jonathan M. 2010. *The Protest Psychosis: How Schizophrenia Became a Black Disease*. Boston: Beacon.

Metzl, Jonathan M., and Anna Kirkland, eds. 2010. *Against Health: How Health Became the New Morality*. New York: NYU Press.

Meyer, Ilan H. 2003. "Prejudice, Social Stress, and Mental Health in Lesbian, Gay, and Bisexual Populations: Conceptual Issues and Research Evidence." *Psychological Bulletin* 129 (5): 674–697.

Meyerowitz, Joanne. 2004. *How Sex Changed: A History of Transsexuality in the United States*. Boston: Harvard University Press.

———. 2008. "AHR Forum: A History of 'Gender.'" *American Historical Review* 113 (5): 1346–1356.

Mohr, Holbrook. 2013. "Illegal Buttocks Injections Kill, Maim U.S. Women." *USA Today*, August 5, 2013. https://www.usatoday.com/story/news/nation/2013/08/05/illegal-buttocks-injections-kill-maim-us-women/2618887/.

Mollow, Anna. 2016. "The Foodscape Argument: When Fatphobia Poses as Radical Social Critique." *Food, Fatness and Fitness* (blog). June 21, 2016. http://foodfatnessfitness.com/2016/06/21/foodscape-argument-fatphobia-poses-radical-social-critique/.

Moraga, Cherríe L. 2000. *Loving in the War Years: Lo Que Nunca Paso Por Sus Labios*. 2nd, expanded ed. Cambridge, MA: South End Press.

Morgan, Kathryn Pauly. 1991. "Women and the Knife: Cosmetic Surgery and the Colonization of Women's Bodies." *Hypatia* 6 (3): 25–53.

Morland, Iain. 2001. "Feminism and Intersexuality: A Response to Myra J. Hird's 'Gender's Nature.'" *Feminist Theory* 2 (3): 362–366.

Morrill, Hannah. 2017. "A Woman Died After Getting CEMENT Butt Injections—Now Her 'Doctor' Is Getting Jail Time." *Allure*, March 29, 2017. https://www.allure.com/story/cement-butt-injections-fake-doctor-jail.

Moten, Fred. 2017. *Black and Blur*. Durham, NC: Duke University Press.

Moynihan, Ray. 2010a. "FDA Advisers to Assess Drug for Low Sexual Desire in Women." *BMJ* 340: c2786.

———. 2010b. "Drug for Low Sexual Desire Carries Significant Harms, FDA Advisers Find." *BMJ* 341: c3339.

Moynihan, Ray, and Alan Cassels. 2006. *Selling Sickness: How the World's Biggest Pharmaceutical Companies Are Turning Us All into Patients*. New York: Nation Books.

Mukherjee, Sy. 2018. "Viagra Anniversary: How Much Pfizer Has Made off the Drug." *Fortune*, March 27, 2018. http://fortune.com/2018/03/27/viagra-anniversary-pfizer/.

Müller, Markus K., Christa Wenger, Marc Schiesser, Pierre-Alain Clavien, and Markus Weber. 2008. "Quality of Life after Bariatric Surgery—A Comparative Study of Laparoscopic Banding vs. Bypass." *Obesity Surgery* 18 (12): 1551–1557.

Muñoz, José Esteban. 1999. *Disidentifications: Queers of Color and the Performance of Politics*. Minneapolis: University of Minnesota Press.

Murad, Mohammad Hassan, Mohamed B. Elamin, Magaly Zumaeta Garcia, Rebecca J. Mullan, Ayman Murad, Patricia J. Erwin, and Victor M. Montori. 2010. "Hormonal Therapy and Sex Reassignment: A Systematic Review and Meta-Analysis of Quality of Life and Psychosocial Outcomes." *Clinical Endocrinology* 72 (2): 214–231.

Murphy, Michelle. 2012. "Pap Smears, Cervical Cancer, and Scales." In *Seizing the Means of Reproduction: Entanglements of Feminism, Health, and Technoscience*, ed. Michelle Murphy, 102–149. Durham, NC: Duke University Press.

Murray, Samantha. 2005. "Doing Politics or Selling Out? Living the Fat Body." *Women's Studies* 34 (3–4): 265–277.

Murray, Samantha, and Nikki Sullivan. 2012. *Somatechnics: Queering the Technologisation of Bodies*. Farnham, UK: Ashgate Publishing, Ltd.

Najmabadi, Afsaneh. 2008. "Transing and Transpassing across Sex-Gender Walls in Iran." *WSQ: Women's Studies Quarterly* 36 (3): 23–42.

———. 2013. *Professing Selves: Transsexuality and Same-Sex Desire in Contemporary Iran*. Durham, NC: Duke University Press.

Namaste, Viviane. 2000. *Invisible Lives: The Erasure of Transsexual and Transgendered People*. Chicago: University of Chicago Press.

———. 2011. *Sex Change, Social Change: Reflections on Identity, Institutions, and Imperialism*. Toronto: Canadian Scholars' Press.

Nappi, Rossella E., Erica Terreno, Ellis Martini, Francesca Albani, Valentina Santamaria, Silvia Tonani, and Franco Polatti. 2010. "Hypoactive Sexual Desire Disorder: Can We Treat It with Drugs?" *Sexual and Relationship Therapy* 25 (3): 264–274.

Narayan, Uma. 2013. *Dislocating Cultures: Identities, Traditions, and Third World Feminism*. New York: Routledge.

Nash, Kate. 2002. "Human Rights for Women: An Argument for 'Deconstructive Equality.'" *Economy and Society* 31 (3): 414–433.

"The National Association to Advance Fat Acceptance." n.d. Accessed August 4, 2016. http://www.naafaonline.com/dev2/index.html.

National Center for Transgender Equality. 2016. "Frequently Asked Questions about Transgender People." https://transequality.org/issues/resources/frequently-asked -questions-about-transgender-people, n.p.

National Research Council. 2007. *Preterm Birth: Causes, Consequences, and Prevention*. ed Richard E. Behrman and Adrienne Stith Butler. Washington, DC: National Academies Press.

National Women's Health Network (NWHN). 2016. "Addyi 1 Year Later: What's the Score?" *NWHN* (blog). August 18, 2016. https://www.nwhn.org/addyi-1-year-later/.

Nelson, Gary. 2011a. "$15K Bond for Accused Fake Doc in Toxic Tush Case." *CBS Miami*, November 24, 2011. http://miami.cbslocal.com/2011/11/24/91050/.

———. 2011b. "New Victim Reveals Fake Doc's Alleged Work." *CBS Miami*, November 28, 2011. http://miami.cbslocal.com/2011/11/28/new-victim-reveals-fake-docs-alleged-work/.

Nelson, Hilde Lindemann, and James Lindemann Nelson. 2013. "Justice in the Allocation of Health Care Resources: A Feminist Account." In *Meaning and Medicine: A*

Reader in the Philosophy of Health Care, ed. James Lindemann Nelson and Hilde Lindemann Nelson, 289. New York: Routledge.

Nelson, James Lindemann. 1996. "Measured Fairness, Situated Justice: Feminist Reflections on Health Care Rationing." *Kennedy Institute of Ethics Journal* 6 (1): 53–68.

———. 2016. "Understanding Transgender and Medically Assisted Gender Transition: Feminism as a Critical Resource." *AMA Journal of Ethics* 18 (11): 1133.

Nestle, M., and M. F. Jacobson. 2000. "Halting the Obesity Epidemic: A Public Health Policy Approach." *Public Health Reports* 115 (1): 12–24.

Nestle, Marion. 2013. *Food Politics: How the Food Industry Influences Nutrition and Health.* Berkeley: University of California Press.

Nettleton, Sarah. 2006. "'I Just Want Permission to Be Ill': Towards a Sociology of Medically Unexplained Symptoms." *Social Science & Medicine* 62 (5): 1167–1178.

Nicholls, Stuart G. 2013. "Standards and Classification: A Perspective on the 'Obesity Epidemic.'" *Social Science & Medicine* 87 (June): 9–15.

Niederdeppe, Jeff, Xiaodong Kuang, Brittney Crock, and Ashley Skelton. 2008. "Media Campaigns to Promote Smoking Cessation among Socioeconomically Disadvantaged Populations: What Do We Know, What Do We Need to Learn, and What Should We Do Now?" *Social Science & Medicine* 67 (9): 1343–1355.

Nielsen, Kim E. 2012. *A Disability History of the United States.* Boston: Beacon.

Nixon, Laura. 2013. "The Right to (Trans) Parent: A Reproductive Justice Approach to Reproductive Rights, Fertility, and Family-Building Issues Facing Transgender People." *William & Mary Journal of Women and the Law* 20: 73.

Noble, Jean Bobby. 2006. *Sons of the Movement: FtMs Risking Incoherence on a Post-Queer Cultural Landscape.* Toronto: Women's Press.

Noone, Jack H., and Christine Stephens. 2008. "Men, Masculine Identities, and Health Care Utilisation." *Sociology of Health & Illness* 30 (5): 711–725.

Norsigian, Judy. 1993. "Women and National Health Care Reform: A Progressive Feminist Agenda." *Journal of Women's Health* 2 (1): 91–94.

Nurnberg, H. George, Paula L. Hensley, Julia R. Heiman, Harry A. Croft, Charles Debattista, and Susan Paine. 2008. "Sildenafil Treatment of Women with Antidepressant-Associated Sexual Dysfunction." *JAMA: The Journal of the American Medical Association* 300 (4): 395–404.

Nygren, Katarina Giritli, Siv Fahlgren, and Anders Johansson. 2015. "(Re)Assembling the 'Normal' in Neoliberal Policy Discourses: Tracing Gender Regimes in the Age of Risk." *Nordic Journal of Social Research* 6: 24–43.

Oaks, Laury. 2001. *Smoking and Pregnancy: The Politics of Fetal Protection.* New Brunswick, NJ: Rutgers University Press.

Obama, Michelle. 2012. "Let's Move! Raising a Healthier Generation of Kids." *Childhood Obesity* 8 (1): 1.

Obeidat, Firas, Hiba Shanti, Ayman Mismar, Nader Albsoul, and Mohammad Al-Qudah. 2015. "The Magnitude of Antral Resection in Laparoscopic Sleeve Gastrectomy and Its Relationship to Excess Weight Loss." *Obesity Surgery* 25 (10): 1928–1932.

O'Brien, Michelle. 2013. "Tracing This Body: Transsexuality, Pharmaceuticals & Capitalism." In *The Transgender Studies Reader 2*, ed. Susan Stryker and Aren Aizura. New York: Routledge.

Oliphant, James. 2011. "Conservatives Dig into Michelle Obama's Anti-Obesity Campaign." *Los Angeles Times*, February 26, 2011. http://articles.latimes.com/2011/feb/26/nation/la-na-michelle-obama-obesity-20110227.

Oliver, J. Eric. 2006. "The Politics of Pathology: How Obesity Became an Epidemic Disease." *Perspectives in Biology and Medicine* 49 (4): 611–627.

Oosterhuis, Harry. 2000. *Stepchildren of Nature: Krafft-Ebing, Psychiatry, and the Making of Sexual Identity*. Chicago: University of Chicago Press.

Orbach, Susie. 1997. *Fat Is a Feminist Issue*. New York: Bbs Pub Corp.

Ordover, Nancy. 2003. *American Eugenics: Race, Queer Anatomy, and the Science of Nationalism*. Minneapolis: University of Minnesota Press.

Padma-Nathan, Harin. 2006. "Sildenafil Citrate (Viagra) Treatment for Erectile Dysfunction: An Updated Profile of Response and Effectiveness." *International Journal of Impotence Research* 18 (5): 423–431.

Padwal, R., S. K. Li, and D. C. W. Lau. 2004. "Long-Term Pharmacotherapy for Obesity and Overweight." *The Cochrane Database of Systematic Reviews*, no. 3: CD004094.

Pascoe, Elizabeth A., and Laura Smart Richman. 2009. "Perceived Discrimination and Health: A Meta-Analytic Review." *Psychological Bulletin* 135 (4): 531–554.

Penney, Tarra L., and Sara F. L. Kirk. 2015. "The Health at Every Size Paradigm and Obesity: Missing Empirical Evidence May Help Push the Reframing Obesity Debate Forward." *American Journal of Public Health* 105 (5): e38–e42.

Petersen, Alan, and Deborah Lupton. 1996. *The New Public Health: Discourses, Knowledges, Strategies*. London: SAGE.

Pfizer. 2010. "VIAGRA U.S. Physician Prescribing Information and U.S. Patient Product Information." http://media.pfizer.com/files/products/uspi_viagra.pdf.

———. n.d. "Erectile Dysfunction Symptoms and Causes." Accessed September 17, 2013. http://www.viagra.com/about-erectile-dysfunction/erectile-dysfunction.aspx.

Philip, Kavita. 2004. *Civilizing Natures: Race, Resources, and Modernity in Colonial South India*. New Brunswick, NJ: Rutgers University Press.

Phillips, Anne. 2010. "What's Wrong with Essentialism?" *Distinktion: Journal of Social Theory* 11(1): 47–60.

Piercy, Marge. 1976. *Woman on the Edge of Time*. New York: Ballantine.

Pinkhasov, R. M., J. Wong, J. Kashanian, M. Lee, D. B. Samadi, M. M. Pinkhasov, and R. Shabsigh. 2010. "Are Men Shortchanged on Health? Perspective on Health Care Utilization and Health Risk Behavior in Men and Women in the United States." *International Journal of Clinical Practice* 64 (4): 475–487.

Pitts-Taylor, Victoria. 2007. *Surgery Junkies: Wellness and Pathology in Cosmetic Culture*. New Brunswick, NJ: Rutgers University Press.

Plemons, Eric D. 2014. "It Is as It Does: Genital Form and Function in Sex Reassignment Surgery." *Journal of Medical Humanities* 35 (1): 37–55.

———. 2017. *The Look of a Woman: Facial Feminization Surgery and the Aims of Trans-Medicine*. Durham, NC: Duke University Press.

Pletcher, Mark J., Stefan G. Kertesz, Michael A. Kohn, and Ralph Gonzales. 2008. "Trends in Opioid Prescribing by Race/Ethnicity for Patients Seeking Care in US Emergency Departments." *JAMA* 299 (1): 70–78.

Pollock, Anne. 2011. "Transforming the Critique of Big Pharma." *BioSocieties* 6 (1): 106–118.

———. 2012. *Medicating Race: Heart Disease and Durable Preoccupations with Difference*. Durham, NC: Duke University Press.

Pollock, Anne, and David S. Jones. 2015. "Coronary Artery Disease and the Contours of Pharmaceuticalization." *Social Science & Medicine* 131 (April): 221–227.

Porter, Roy. 2004. *Blood and Guts: A Short History of Medicine*. New York: W. W. Norton.

"Potential Candidates for Bariatric Surgery." n.d. National Institute of Diabetes and Digestive and Kidney Diseases. Accessed February 21, 2017. https://www.niddk.nih.gov/health-information/health-topics/weight-control/bariatric-surgery/Pages/potential-candidates.aspx.

Potts, Annie, Nicola Gavey, Victoria M. Grace, and Tiina Vares. 2003. "The Downside of Viagra: Women's Experiences and Concerns." *Sociology of Health & Illness* 25 (7): 697–719.

Potts, Annie, Victoria Grace, Nicola Gavey, and Tiina Vares. 2004. "'Viagra Stories': Challenging 'Erectile Dysfunction.'" *Social Science & Medicine* 59 (3): 489–499.

Potts, Annie, Victoria M. Grace, Tiina Vares, and Nicola Gavey. 2006. "'Sex for Life'? Men's Counter-Stories on 'Erectile Dysfunction', Male Sexuality and Ageing." *Sociology of Health & Illness* 28 (3): 306–329.

Preciado, Paul B. 2013. *Testo Junkie: Sex, Drugs, and Biopolitics in the Pharmacopornographic Era*. New York: The Feminist Press at CUNY.

Preves, Sharon E. 2003. *Intersex and Identity: The Contested Self*. New Brunswick, NJ: Rutgers University Press.

Price, Kimala. 2011. "What Is Reproductive Justice? How Women of Color Activists Are Redefining the Pro-Choice Paradigm." *Meridians: Feminism, Race, Transnationalism* 10 (2): 42–65.

Prince, S. A. 2009. "A Population Health Approach to Obesity in Canada—Putting the Problem Back into Context." *Transdisciplinary Studies in Population Health Series* 1 (1): 22–33.

Proctor, Robert. 1988. *Racial Hygiene: Medicine under the Nazis*. Boston, MA: Harvard University Press.

Prosser, Jay. 1998. *Second Skins*. New York: Columbia University Press.

Provencher, Véronique, Catherine Bégin, Angelo Tremblay, Lyne Mongeau, Sonia Boivin, and Simone Lemieux. 2007. "Short-Term Effects of a 'Health-At-Every-Size' Approach on Eating Behaviors and Appetite Ratings." *Obesity* 15 (4): 957–966.

Provencher, Véronique, Catherine Bégin, Angelo Tremblay, Lyne Mongeau, Louise Corneau, Sylvie Dodin, Sonia Boivin, and Simone Lemieux. 2009. "Health-at-Every-Size and Eating Behaviors: 1-Year Follow-up Results of a Size Acceptance Intervention." *Journal of the American Dietetic Association* 109 (11): 1854–1861.

Puar, Jasbir K. 2007. *Terrorist Assemblages: Homonationalism in Queer Times*. Durham, NC: Duke University Press.

———. 2015. "Bodies with New Organs: Becoming Trans, Becoming Disabled." *Social Text* 33 (3124): 45–73.

Puhl, R., and K. D. Brownell. 2001. "Bias, Discrimination, and Obesity." *Obesity Research* 9 (12): 788–805.

Puhl, R. M., T. Andreyeva, and K. D. Brownell. 2008. "Perceptions of Weight Discrimination: Prevalence and Comparison to Race and Gender Discrimination in America." *International Journal of Obesity* 32 (6): 992–1000.

Purdy, Laura. 2001. "Medicalization, Medical Necessity, and Feminist Medicine." *Bioethics* 15 (3): 248–261.

Puzziferri, Nancy, Thomas B. Roshek, Helen G. Mayo, Ryan Gallagher, Steven H. Belle, and Edward H. Livingston. 2014. "Long-Term Follow-up After Bariatric Surgery: A Systematic Review." *JAMA* 312 (9): 934–942.

Rabiner, Stephanie. 2012. "Are Silicone Injections Legal?" Findlaw. January 10, 2012. http://blogs.findlaw.com/injured/2012/01/are-silicone-injections-legal.html.

Rabinow, Paul, and Nikolas Rose. 2006. "Biopower Today." *BioSocieties* 1 (2): 195–217.

Race, Kane. 2009. *Pleasure Consuming Medicine: The Queer Politics of Drugs*. Durham, NC: Duke University Press.

Rapp, Rayna. 2004. *Testing Women, Testing the Fetus: The Social Impact of Amniocentesis in America*. New York: Routledge.

Raymond, Diane. 1999. "'Fatal Practices': A Feminist Analysis of Physician-Assisted Suicide and Euthanasia." *Hypatia* 14 (2): 1–25.

Raymond, Janice G. 1974. *The Transsexual Empire: The Making of the She-Male*. Boston: Beacon Press.

Reilly, Niamh. 2007. "Cosmopolitan Feminism and Human Rights." *Hypatia* 22 (4): 180–198.

Reis, Elizabeth. 2009. *Bodies in Doubt: An American History of Intersex*. Baltimore: Johns Hopkins University Press.

"Reproductive Justice." n.d. Sister Song, Inc. Accessed April 24, 2017. http://sistersong.net/reproductive-justice/.

"REtransition." n.d. REtransition. Accessed April 20, 2017. http://retransition.org/.

Riessman, C. K. 1983. "Women and Medicalization: A New Perspective." *Social Policy* 14 (1): 3–18.

Riley, Wayne J. 2012. "Health Disparities: Gaps in Access, Quality and Affordability of Medical Care." *Transactions of the American Clinical and Climatological Association* 123: 167–174.

Roberts, Celia. 2006. "'What Can I Do to Help Myself?' Somatic Individuality and Contemporary Hormonal Bodies." *Science & Technology Studies* 19 (2): 54–76.

Roberts, Dorothy E. 1993. "Racism and Patriarchy in the Meaning of Motherhood." *The American University Journal of Gender, Social Policy & the Law* 1 (1): 1–38.

———. 1999. *Killing the Black Body: Race, Reproduction, and the Meaning of Liberty*. New York: Vintage.

———. 2008. "Is Race-Based Medicine Good for Us? African American Approaches to Race, Biomedicine, and Equality." *Journal of Law, Medicine & Ethics* 36 (3): 537–545.

———. 2015. "Reproductive Justice, Not Just Rights." *Dissent Magazine*. https://www.dissentmagazine.org/issue/fall-2015.

Robertson, Ann. 2000. "Embodying Risk, Embodying Political Rationality: Women's Accounts of Risks for Breast Cancer." *Health, Risk & Society* 2 (2): 219–235.

Robertson, Scott Michael. 2009. "Neurodiversity, Quality of Life, and Autistic Adults: Shifting Research and Professional Focuses onto Real-Life Challenges." *Disability Studies Quarterly* 30 (1).

Roehling, Mark V., Patricia V. Roehling, and Shaun Pichler. 2007. "The Relationship between Body Weight and Perceived Weight-Related Employment Discrimination: The Role of Sex and Race." *Journal of Vocational Behavior* 71 (2): 300–318.

Rose, Nikolas S. 2007. *Politics of Life Itself: Biomedicine, Power, and Subjectivity in the Twenty-First Century.* Princeton, NJ: Princeton University Press.

Ross, Loretta, and Rickie Solinger. 2017. *Reproductive Justice: An Introduction.* Berkeley: University of California Press.

Roth, Louise Marie, and Megan M. Henley. 2012. "Unequal Motherhood: Racial-Ethnic and Socioeconomic Disparities in Cesarean Sections in the United States." *Social Problems* 59 (2): 207–227.

Rothenberg, Bess. 2003. "'We Don't Have Time for Social Change' Cultural Compromise and the Battered Woman Syndrome." *Gender & Society* 17 (5): 771–787.

Rotondi, Nooshin Khobzi, Greta R. Bauer, Kyle Scanlon, Matthias Kaay, Robb Travers, and Anna Travers. 2013. "Nonprescribed Hormone Use and Self-Performed Surgeries: 'Do-It-Yourself' Transitions in Transgender Communities in Ontario, Canada." *American Journal of Public Health* 103 (10): 1830–1836.

Rubin, David A. 2012. "'An Unnamed Blank That Craved a Name': A Genealogy of Intersex as Gender." *Signs* 37 (4): 883–908.

———. 2015. "Provincializing Intersex: US Intersex Activism, Human Rights, and Transnational Body Politics." *Frontiers: A Journal of Women Studies* 36 (3): 51–83.

———. 2017. *Intersex Matters: Biomedical Embodiment, Gender Regulation, and Transnational Activism.* Albany: State University of New York Press.

Rubin, Gayle. 1984. "Thinking Sex: Notes for a Radical Theory of the Politics of Sexuality." In *Pleasure and Danger: Exploring Female Sexuality,* ed. Carole S. Vance. Boston: Routledge and Kegan Paul.

Rucker, Diana, Raj Padwal, Stephanie K. Li, Cintia Curioni, and David C. W. Lau. 2007. "Long Term Pharmacotherapy for Obesity and Overweight: Updated Meta-Analysis." *BMJ* 335 (7631): 1194–1199.

Rucovsky, Martin De Mauro. 2015. "Trans* Necropolitics. Gender Identity Law in Argentina." *Sexualidad, Salud y Sociedad; Rio de Janeiro,* no. 20 (August): 10–27.

Ruhl, Sarah. 2010. *In the Next Room.* New York: Theatre Communications Group.

Runswick-Cole, Katherine. 2014. "'Us' and 'Them': The Limits and Possibilities of a 'Politics of Neurodiversity' in Neoliberal Times." *Disability & Society* 29 (7): 1117–1129.

Russell, Jill, Deborah Swinglehurst, and Trisha Greenhalgh. 2014. "'Cosmetic Boob Jobs' or Evidence-Based Breast Surgery: An Interpretive Policy Analysis of the Rationing of 'Low Value' Treatments in the English National Health Service." *BMC Health Services Research* 14: 413.

Sabin, Janice A., Brian. A. Nosek, Anthony G. Greenwald, and Frederick P. Rivara. 2009. "Physicians' Implicit and Explicit Attitudes About Race by MD Race, Ethnicity, and Gender." *Journal of Health Care for the Poor and Underserved* 20 (3): 896–913.

Sainsbury, Amanda, and Phillipa Hay. 2014. "Call for an Urgent Rethink of the 'Health at Every Size' Concept." *Journal of Eating Disorders* 2 (March): 8.

Salamon, Gayle. 2010. *Assuming a Body: Transgender and Rhetorics of Materiality.* New York: Columbia University Press.

Sandahl, Carrie. 2003. "Queering the Crip or Cripping the Queer? Intersections of Queer and Crip Identities in Solo Autobiographical Performance." *GLQ: A Journal of Lesbian and Gay Studies* 9 (1): 25–56.

Sastre, Alexandra. 2014. "Hottentot in the Age of Reality TV: Sexuality, Race, and Kim Kardashian's Visible Body." *Celebrity Studies* 5 (1–2): 123–137.

Savulescu, Julian. 2001. "Procreative Beneficence: Why We Should Select the Best Children." *Bioethics* 15 (5–6): 413–426.

Savulescu, Julian, and Guy Kahane. 2009. "The Moral Obligation to Create Children with the Best Chance of the Best Life." *Bioethics* 23 (5): 274–290.

Sawicki, Jana. 1991. *Disciplining Foucault: Feminism, Power, and the Body.* New York: Routledge.

Saxton, Marsha. 2013. "Disability Rights and Selective Abortion." In *The Disability Studies Reader*, ed. Lennard J. Davis, 4th ed., 87–99. New York: Routledge.

Scheper-Hughes, Nancy, and Margaret M. Lock. 1987. "The Mindful Body: A Prolegomenon to Future Work in Medical Anthropology." *Medical Anthropology Quarterly* 1 (1): 6–41.

Schweik, Susan M. 2009. *The Ugly Laws: Disability in Public.* New York: NYU Press.

Sedgwick, Eve Kosofsky. 1990. "Axiomatic." In *Epistemology of the Closet*, xi. Berkeley: University of California Press.

Sennott, Shannon L. 2010. "Gender Disorder as Gender Oppression: A Transfeminist Approach to Rethinking the Pathologization of Gender Non-Conformity." *Women & Therapy* 34 (1–2): 93–113.

Serano, Julia. 2007. *Whipping Girl: A Transsexual Woman on Sexism and the Scapegoating of Femininity.* Annotated ed. Emeryville, CA: Seal Press.

Sexton, Jared. 2008. *Amalgamation Schemes: Antiblackness and the Critique of Multiracialism.* Minneapolis: University of Minnesota Press.

Siebers, Tobin Anthony. 2008. *Disability Theory.* Ann Arbor: University of Michigan Press.

———. 2013. "Disability and the Theory of Complex Embodiment—For Identity Politics in a New Register." In *The Disability Studies Reader*, ed. Lennard Davis, 4th ed. New York: Routledge.

Sifferlin, Alexandra. 2017. "Gender Confirmation Surgery Is on the Rise in the U.S." *Time*, May 22, 2017. http://time.com/4787914/transgender-gender-confirmation-surgery/.

Silver, Anne E. 2013. "An Offer You Can't Refuse: Coercing Consent to Surgery through the Medicalization of Gender Identity." *Columbia Journal of Gender and Law* 26: 488.

Skinner, Daniel. 2012. "The Politics of Medical Necessity in American Abortion Debates." *Politics & Gender* 8 (1): 1–24.

Smith, Andrea. 2005. "Beyond Pro-Choice Versus Pro-Life: Women of Color and Reproductive Justice." *NWSA Journal* 17 (1): 119–140.

Smith, S. E. 2014. "Not Your Good Fatty: HAES and Disability." *Disability Intersections* (blog). June 2, 2014. http://disabilityintersections.com/2014/06/453/.

Snorton, C. Riley, and Jin Haritaworn. 2013. "Trans Necropolitics: A Transnational Reflection on Violence, Death, and the Trans of Color Afterlife." In *The Transgender Studies Reader 2*, ed. Susan Stryker and Aren Aizura, 66–75. New York: Routledge.

Spade, Dean. 2003. "Resisting Medicine, Re/Modeling Gender." *Berkeley Women's Law Journal* 18: 15–39.

———. 2011. *Normal Life: Administrative Violence, Critical Trans Politics and the Limits of Law.* Brooklyn, NY: South End Press.

Sparrow, Robert. 2011. "A Not-so-New Eugenics: Harris and Savulescu on Human Enhancement." *The Hastings Center Report* 41 (1): 32–42.

———. 2013a. "Gender Eugenics? The Ethics of PGD for Intersex Conditions." *American Journal of Bioethics* 13 (10): 29–38.

———. 2013b. "Queerin' the PGD Clinic: Human Enhancement and the Future of Bodily Diversity." *Journal of Medical Humanities* 34: 177–196.

Stone, Sandy. 1992. "The Empire Strikes Back: A Posttranssexual Manifesto." *Camera Obscura* 10 (2, 29): 150–176.

"Stop Trans Pathologization—2012." n.d. Accessed April 17, 2017. http://www.stp2012 .info/old/en/objectives.

Stoppard, Janet. 2014. *Understanding Depression: Feminist Social Constructionist Approaches.* New York: Routledge.

STP—International Campaign Stop Trans Pathologization. 2016. "Press Release: International Day of Action for Trans Depathologization 2016." http://www.stp2012.info /STP_Press_Release_October2016.pdf.

Stryker, Susan. 2009. *Transgender History.* Berkeley: Seal Press.

———. 2012. "De/Colonizing Transgender Studies of China." In *Transgender China*, ed. Howard Chiang, 287–292. New York: Palgrave Macmillan US.

Stryker, Susan, and Nikki Sullivan. 2009. "King's Member, Queen's Body: Transsexual Surgery, Self-Demand Amputation and the Somatechnics of Sovereign Power." In *Somatechnics: Queering the Technologisation of Bodies*, ed. Samantha Murray and Nikki Sullivan, 49–64. Farnham, UK: Ashgate Publishing, Ltd.

Styperek, Andrew, Stephanie Bayers, Michael Beer, and Kenneth Beer. 2013. "Nonmedical-Grade Injections of Permanent Fillers." *Journal of Clinical and Aesthetic Dermatology* 6 (4): 22–29.

Suess, Amets, Karine Espineira, and Pau Crego Walters. 2014. "Depathologization." *TSQ: Transgender Studies Quarterly* 1 (1–2): 73–77.

Sugg, N., and T. Inui. 1992. "Primary Care Physicians' Response to Domestic Violence: Opening Pandora's Box." *JAMA* 267 (23): 3157–3160.

Sullivan, Nikki. 2014. "Somatechnics." *TSQ: Transgender Studies Quarterly* 1 (1–2): 187–190.

Swearingen, Sean G., and Jeffrey D. Klausner. 2005. "Sildenafil Use, Sexual Risk Behavior, and Risk for Sexually Transmitted Diseases, Including HIV Infection." *American Journal of Medicine* 118 (6): 571–577.

Sweet, Paige L. 2014. "'Every Bone of My Body:' Domestic Violence and the Diagnostic Body." *Social Science & Medicine* 122 (December): 44–52.

Tanne, Janice Hopkins. 2010. "Michelle Obama Launches Programme to Combat US Childhood Obesity." *BMJ: British Medical Journal (Online)* 340.

Tate, Allison. 2017. "Asia Kate Dillon Explains Gender-Nonbinary to Ellen." *The Advocate*, March 21, 2017. http://www.advocate.com/arts-entertainment/2017/3/21/asia -kate-dillon-explains-gender-nonbinary-ellen.

Teghtsoonian, Katherine. 2009. "Depression and Mental Health in Neoliberal Times: A Critical Analysis of Policy and Discourse." *Social Science & Medicine* 69 (1): 28–35.

Temple Newhook, Julia, Deborah Gregory, and Laurie Twells. 2015. "'Fat Girls' and 'Big Guys': Gendered Meanings of Weight Loss Surgery." *Sociology of Health & Illness* 37 (5): 653–667.

Terry, Jennifer. 1999. *An American Obsession: Science, Medicine, and Homosexuality in Modern Society.* Chicago: University of Chicago Press.

———. 2009. "Significant Injury: War, Medicine, and Empire in Claudia's Case." *WSQ: Women's Studies Quarterly* 37 (1): 200–225.

Thaler, Richard H., and Cass R. Sunstein. 2009. *Nudge: Improving Decisions about Health, Wealth, and Happiness.* Rev. and expanded ed. New York: Penguin Books.

"Think Before You Pink." n.d. Accessed December 21, 2018. http://thinkbeforeyoupink .org/past-campaigns/.

Thompson, L. E., J. R. Barnett, and J. R. Pearce. 2009. "Scared Straight? Fear-Appeal Anti-Smoking Campaigns, Risk, Self-Efficacy and Addiction." *Health, Risk & Society* 11 (2): 181–196.

Throsby, Karen. 2007. "'How Could You Let Yourself Get Like That?' Stories of the Origins of Obesity in Accounts of Weight Loss Surgery." *Social Science & Medicine* 65 (8): 1561–1571.

———. 2008. "Happy Re-Birthday: Weight Loss Surgery and the 'New Me.'" *Body & Society* 14 (1): 117–133.

Tiefer, Leonore. 2003. "The Pink Viagra Story: We Have the Drug, but What's the Disease?" *Radical Philosophy* 121 (October): 2–5.

———. 2004. *Sex Is Not a Natural Act & Other Essays.* 2nd ed. Boulder, CO: Westview Press.

———. 2006. "Female Sexual Dysfunction: A Case Study of Disease Mongering and Activist Resistance." *PLoS Med* 3 (4): e178.

Titchkosky, Tanya. 2011. *The Question of Access: Disability, Space, Meaning.* Toronto: University of Toronto Press, Scholarly Publishing Division.

Tosh, Jemma. 2016. *Psychology and Gender Dysphoria: Feminist and Transgender Perspectives.* New York: Routledge.

Tower, Marion. 2007. "Intimate Partner Violence and the Health Care Response: A Postmodern Critique." *Health Care for Women International* 28 (5): 438–452.

Tyler, Meagan. 2008. "No Means Yes? Perpetuating Myths in the Sexological Construction of Women's Desire." *Women & Therapy* 32 (1): 40–50.

"Types of Bariatric Surgery." n.d. National Institute of Diabetes and Digestive and Kidney Diseases. Accessed February 22, 2017. https://www.niddk.nih.gov/health -information/health-topics/weight-control/bariatric-surgery/Pages/types.aspx.

U.S. Department of Health and Human Services. n.d. "Access to Health Services." https://www.healthypeople.gov/2020/topics-objectives/topic/Access-to-Health -Services/national-snapshot.

U.S. Department of Health and Human Services and U.S. Department of Agriculture. 2015. *2015–2020 Dietary Guidelines for Americans.* 8th edition. Available at http:// health.gov/dietaryguidelines/2015/guidelines/.

Ussher, Jane M. 2003. "The Role of Premenstrual Dysphoric Disorder in the Subjectification of Women." *Journal of Medical Humanities* 24 (1–2): 131–146.

———. 2010. "Are We Medicalizing Women's Misery? A Critical Review of Women's Higher Rates of Reported Depression." *Feminism & Psychology* 20 (1): 9–35.

Valentine, David. 2007. *Imagining Transgender: An Ethnography of a Category.* Durham, NC: Duke University Press.

———. 2012. "Sue E. Generous: Toward a Theory of Non-Transexuality." *Feminist Studies* 38 (1): 185–211.

Vares, Tiina, and Virginia Braun. 2006. "Spreading the Word, but What Word Is That? Viagra and Male Sexuality in Popular Culture." *Sexualities* 9 (3): 315–332.

Vipond, Evan. 2015. "Resisting Transnormativity: Challenging the Medicalization and Regulation of Trans Bodies." *Theory in Action* 8 (2): 21–44.

Waites, Matthew. 2009. "Critique of 'Sexual Orientation' and 'Gender Identity' in Human Rights Discourse: Global Queer Politics beyond the Yogyakarta Principles." *Contemporary Politics* 15 (1): 137–156.

Wallace, Amy E., Yinong Young-Xu, David Hartley, and William B. Weeks. 2010. "Racial, Socioeconomic, and Rural–Urban Disparities in Obesity-Related Bariatric Surgery." *Obesity Surgery* 20 (10): 1354–1360.

Wann, Marilyn. 2009. "Foreword: Fat Studies: An Invitation to Revolution." In *The Fat Studies Reader*, ed. Esther Rothblum and Sondra Solovay, xi. New York: NYU Press.

Warholm, Christine, Aud Marie Øien, and Målfrid Råheim. 2014. "The Ambivalence of Losing Weight after Bariatric Surgery." *International Journal of Qualitative Studies on Health and Well-Being* 9 (1): 22876.

Warner, Michael, ed. 1993. *Fear of a Queer Planet: Queer Politics and Social Theory.* Minneapolis: University of Minnesota Press.

———. 2000. *The Trouble with Normal: Sex, Politics, and the Ethics of Queer Life.* Boston: Harvard University Press.

Washington, Harriet A. 2006. *Medical Apartheid: The Dark History of Medical Experimentation on Black Americans from Colonial Times to the Present.* New York: Harlem Moon Broadway Books.

Weaver, A. Charlotta, Tosha B. Wetterneck, Chad T. Whelan, and Keiki Hinami. 2015. "A Matter of Priorities? Exploring the Persistent Gender Pay Gap in Hospital Medicine." *Journal of Hospital Medicine* 10 (8): 486–490.

Weinand, Jamie D., and Joshua D. Safer. 2015. "Hormone Therapy in Transgender Adults Is Safe with Provider Supervision; A Review of Hormone Therapy Sequelae for Transgender Individuals." *Journal of Clinical & Translational Endocrinology* 2 (2): 55–60.

Welsh, Talia. 2011. "Healthism and the Bodies of Women: Pleasure and Discipline in the War against Obesity." *Journal of Feminist Scholarship*, no. 1: 33–48.

Wendell, Susan. 1989. "Toward a Feminist Theory of Disability." *Hypatia* 4 (2): 104–124.

———. 2013. *The Rejected Body: Feminist Philosophical Reflections on Disability.* New York: Routledge.

White, Francis Ray. 2012. "Fat, Queer, Dead: 'Obesity' and the Death Drive." *Somatechnics* 2 (1): 1–17.

Wiegman, Robyn. 2017. "Sex and Negativity; or, What Queer Theory Has for You." *Cultural Critique* 95 (1): 219–243.

Willard, Barbara E. 2005. "Feminist Interventions in Biomedical Discourse: An Analysis of the Rhetoric of Integrative Medicine." *Women's Studies in Communication* 28 (1): 115–148.

Williams, Cristan. 2016. "Radical Inclusion: Recounting the Trans Inclusive History of Radical Feminism." *TSQ: Transgender Studies Quarterly* 3 (1–2): 254–258.

Wilson, Elizabeth A. 2004. *Psychosomatic: Feminism and the Neurological Body.* Durham, NC: Duke University Press.

———. 2006. "The Work of Antidepressants: Preliminary Notes on How to Build an Alliance between Feminism and Psychopharmacology." *BioSocieties* 1 (1): 125–131.

———. 2015. *Gut Feminism.* Durham, NC: Duke University Press.

Wilson, Fiona, Christine Ingleton, Merryn Gott, and Clare Gardiner. 2014. "Autonomy and Choice in Palliative Care: Time for a New Model?" *Journal of Advanced Nursing* 70 (5): 1020–1029.

Wolf, Naomi. 2002. *The Beauty Myth: How Images of Beauty Are Used against Women.* Reprint ed. New York: Harper Perennial.

Wolf, Susan M. 1996. "Gender, Feminism, and Death: Physician-Assisted Suicide and Euthanasia." In *Feminism and Bioethics: Beyond Reproduction,* ed Susan M. Wolf. 287–317. New York: Oxford University Press.

Wolpe, P. R. 2002. "Treatment, Enhancement, and the Ethics of Neurotherapeutics." *Brain and Cognition* 50 (3): 387–395.

Woods, Carly S. 2013. "Repunctuated Feminism: Marketing Menstrual Suppression through the Rhetoric of Choice." *Women's Studies in Communication* 36 (3): 267–287.

Woolfolk, Robert L., and Rachel H. Wasserman. 2005. "Count No One Happy: Eudaimonia and Positive Psychology." *Journal of Theoretical and Philosophical Psychology* 25 (1): 81–90.

The Working Group on a New View of Women's Sexual Problems. n.d. "The New View Manifesto—A New View of Women's Sexual Problems." New View Campaign. Accessed September 1, 2011. http://www.newviewcampaign.org/manifesto1.asp.

Worth, Tammy. 2010. "Is the Fat Acceptance Movement Bad for Our Health?" *CNN .com*, January 6, 2010. http://www.cnn.com/2010/HEALTH/01/06/fat.acceptance /index.html.

Yancey, Antronette K., Joanne Leslie, and Emily K. Abel. 2006. "Obesity at the Crossroads: Feminist and Public Health Perspectives." *Signs* 31 (2): 425–443.

Young, Iris Marion. 2002. *Inclusion and Democracy.* Oxford, UK: Oxford University Press.

———. 2005. *On Female Body Experience: "Throwing Like a Girl" and Other Essays.* Oxford, UK: Oxford University Press.

Young, Jessica, and Lisette Burrows. 2013. "Finding the 'Self' after Weight Loss Surgery: Two Women's Experiences." *Feminism & Psychology* 23 (4): 498–516.

Yuval-Davis, Nira. 1993. "Beyond Difference: Women and Coalition Politics." *Making Connections: Women's Studies, Women's Movements, Women's Lives,* ed. Mary Kennedy, Cathy Lubelska, and Val Walsh, 3–10. London: Taylor and Francis.

Zerilli, Linda M. G. 2005. *Feminism and the Abyss of Freedom.* Chicago: University of Chicago Press.

Zhang, Husen, John K. DiBaise, Andrea Zuccolo, Dave Kudrna, Michele Braidotti, Yeisoo Yu, Prathap Parameswaran, et al. 2009. "Human Gut Microbiota in Obesity and after Gastric Bypass." *Proceedings of the National Academy of Sciences* 106 (7): 2365–2370.

Zucker, Kenneth J. 2010. "The DSM Diagnostic Criteria for Gender Identity Disorder in Children." *Archives of Sexual Behavior* 39 (2): 477–498.

Index

About the Author

Kristina Gupta is an assistant professor of women's, gender, and sexuality studies at Wake Forest University. Her interests include contemporary asexual identities and gender, health, and science. She is coeditor of *Queer Feminist Science Studies* (2017) and the author of numerous articles, including "Compulsory Sexuality: Evaluating an Emerging Concept" (2015), in *Signs*.